WEIGHT LOSS

WOMEN OVER 50

Embracing Vitality, Defying Age, and Rediscovering Your Best Self

ZAZABOR GURU

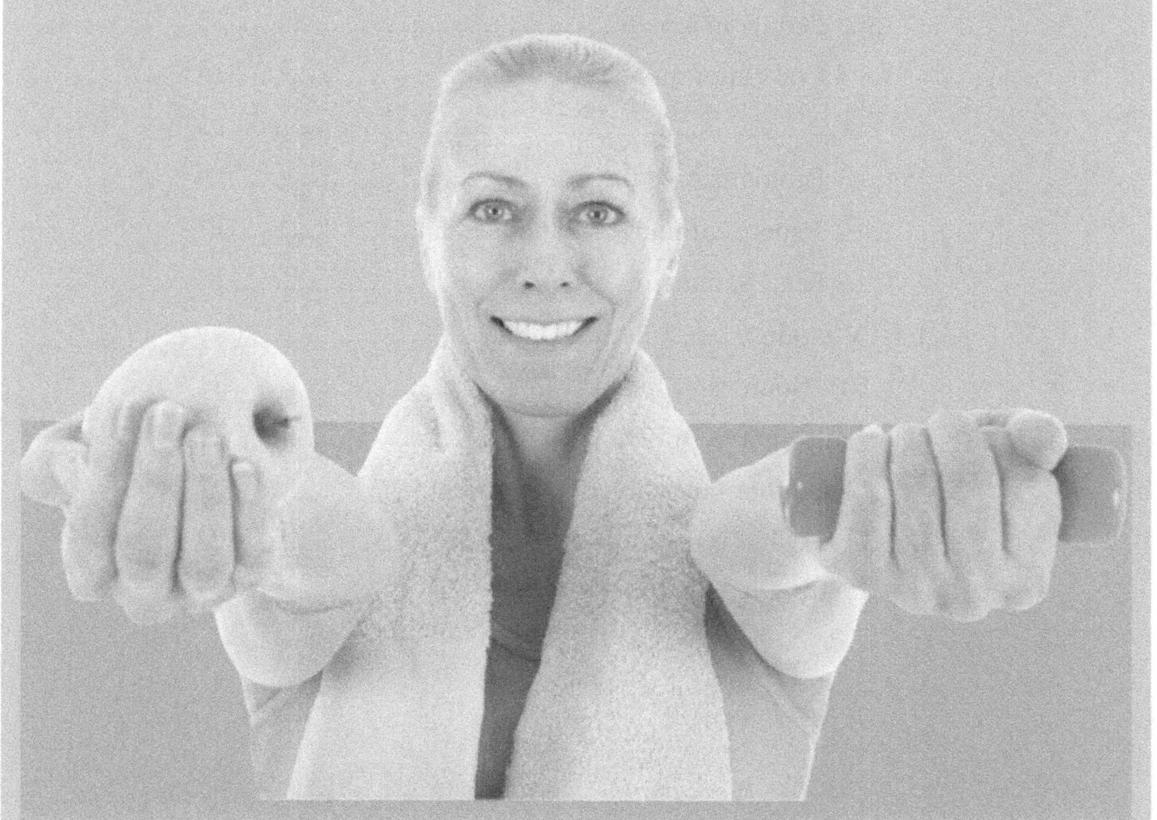

Table of Contents

Introduction

Gone are the days when the human race had to struggle to get a mouthful for their core survival. For the last few centuries - especially after the Industrial Revolution - things have turned out to be nothing but a blessing. People around the world - barring the Arctic and the Antarctic regions, and some parts of Africa - are enjoying the bounty of nature to their heart's content. Getting the food on your dining table has become a task indeed as easy as saying than doing so. All such flexibility, however, has taken its toll on human health. The diversity of food options, along with its richness in preparations, have whet the appetite of not only the gut but also the eyes. Consequently, people are just wolfing the whopping food delicacy. Even if we have the cutting-edge technology at our disposal, the modern science is still feeble in winning the battle against aging smoothly. In fact, it seems we have not been able to shed our ancestral genetic legacy entirely despite the onslaught of consuming artificial edibles. In such a delicate landscape enters the female sex. Although women's genetic resilience is a phenomenon on its own right, their susceptibility to the modern-day lifestyle is equally intriguing. While their seemingly fragile composition can withstand so many rough patches in their physical transformations throughout their life, they seem to be cajoled by the nature's diabolical forces into giving up at a certain age - usually after 50. With a host of complications knocking at the door - in reality banging the door thunderously - they conspicuously become a slave of one particular health hazard - obesity. This silent assassin - it dawns on us - is on a mission to not only agonize the aging XX chromosome bearers, it appears to be bent on wiping out this charming population group, who can enrich the experience of life of other population group with their acquired knowledge and insight. Thus, it is an obligation for us to explore why and how this epidemic has engulfed this population group and how to address this issue with pragmatic prudence.

Chapter 1: Food - our Identity

It is a cliché that life on earth has never been easy. In fact, our modern-day life is the culmination of so many events and variables and their complex combination that even the best of intellectuals would be easily overwhelmed and exasperated. Nevertheless, it does not matter how complicated this survival track record has been for the human race, it primarily survived and sustained on one single component - food. Our present discussion also evolves around this very concept: how food has created such an intricate game puzzle that we have become nothing but mere chess pieces within this setting. Therefore, our discussion would be hitting upon the elaborate details of food and its impact on human health.

1.1 But what is Food?

Well, any substance ingested by an organism for nutritional support is considered food. Food items are predominantly derived from plants, animals, or fungi and comprise vital nutrients including carbohydrates, lipids, proteins, vitamins, and minerals. The substance is assimilated by the cells of an organism after being ingested, for the purposes of providing energy, sustaining life, or promoting growth.

Diverse animal species have developed distinct dietary behaviors to meet the energy demands of their metabolisms and to occupy particular ecological niches in particular geographic regions. Omnivorous Homo sapiens are exceptionally versatile and have acclimated to procure sustenance in numerous ecosystems. For the most part, cooking is how humans prepare sustenance for consumption. The industrial food industry, which produces food via intensive agriculture and distributes it via complex food processing and distribution systems, provides the majority of the energy required for food.

1.2 classification of Food

Now, the term "definition and classification" refers to the process of clearly defining and categorizing something. Food refers to any substance that is ingested by an organism to give nourishment and fuel. Animals can take feed in its raw, processed, or formulated form orally for the purposes of growth, health, or enjoyment.

Food primarily consists of water, fats, proteins, and carbs. Food contains minerals, such as salts, and organic molecules, such as vitamins. Plants, algae, and certain microbes employ sunlight to synthesize a portion of their own nutrition. Water is present in numerous food items and is considered a distinct type of food. Water and fiber have modest caloric densities, but fat is the most calorically dense component.

Certain inorganic elements, which are not related to food, are necessary for the proper functioning of plants and animals. Human food can be categorized using many criteria, such as its composition or the methods used in its preparation. The quantity and constitution of dietary categories may differ. The majority of systems consist of four fundamental categories that delineate their source and their nutritional role: The food groups include Vegetables and Fruit, Cereals and Bread, Dairy, and Meat.

Research examining the quality of diets categorize food items into many groups, including whole grains/cereals, refined grains/cereals, vegetables, fruits, nuts, legumes, eggs, dairy products, fish, red meat, processed meat, and sugar-sweetened beverages.

The Food and Agriculture Organization and World Health Organization employ a classification system consisting of nineteen categories for food: cereals, roots, pulses and nuts, milk, eggs, fish and shellfish, meat, insects, vegetables, fruits, fats and oils, sweets and sugars, spices and condiments, beverages, foods for nutritional purposes, food additives, composite dishes, and savory snacks.

Humans are omnivorous, deriving food from a variety of sources including vegetables, fruits, cooked meat, milk, eggs, mushrooms, and seaweed. Cereal grains are a fundamental source of sustenance, supplying more food energy globally than any other crop kind. Corn (maize), wheat, and rice collectively contribute to 87% of global grain production. Approximately 55 percent of the global crop production is allocated for human consumption, while 36 percent is dedicated to animal feed and 9 percent is utilized for biofuel production. Fungi and bacteria are employed in the production of fermented foods such as bread, wine, cheese, and yogurt.

1.3 Foods derived from plants

Plants are classified as food sources into seeds, fruits, vegetables, legumes, grains, and nuts. Botanically characterized fruits such as the tomato, squash, pepper, and eggplant, as well as seeds such as peas, are often classified as vegetables. Food is considered fruit if the part eaten is derived from the reproductive tissue, which includes seeds, nuts, and grains. Fruits are generally considered the remnants of botanically specified fruits after grains, nuts, seeds, and fruits utilized as vegetables have been removed. Grains are seeds that humans eat or harvest. Cereal grains (oats, wheat, rice, corn, barley, rye, sorghum, and millet) are members of the Poaceae (grass) family, whereas pulses are members of the Fabaceae (legume) family.

Whole grains are foods that have all of the original seed's components (bran, germ, and endosperm). Nuts are dry fruits that are distinguished by their woody shell. Stone fruits (cherries and peaches), pome fruits (apples, pears), berries (blackberry, strawberry), citrus (oranges, lemon), melons (watermelon, cantaloupe), Mediterranean fruits (grapes, fig), and tropical fruits (banana, pineapple) are the different types of fleshy fruits. Vegetables include any additional edible portion of the plant, such as roots, stems, leaves, flowers, bark, or the entire plant. Root vegetables (potatoes and carrots), bulbs (onion family), blossoms (cauliflower and broccoli), leaf vegetables (spinach and lettuce), and stem vegetables (celery and asparagus) are examples of these.

Plants' glucose, protein, and fat content varies greatly. Carbohydrates are mostly starch, fructose, glucose, and other sugars. With the exception of vitamin D and vitamin B12, most vitamins are found in plants. Minerals can also be abundant or scarce. Fruit can include up to 90% water, a high level of simple sugars that contribute to its sweet taste, and a high quantity of vitamin C.

Vegetables are high in carbohydrate, potassium, dietary fiber, folate, and vitamins while being low in fat and calories when compared to fleshy fruit (excluding bananas). Grains are primarily starch-based, whereas nuts are abundant in protein, fiber, vitamin E, and B. Seeds are a useful source of food for animals since they are plentiful and include fiber and healthy fats like omega-3 fats.

 Certain nutrients' bioavailability can be increased or decreased by complex chemical interactions. Some carbohydrates and vitamins can be inhibited by phytates. Humans consume thousands of plant species; there may be as many as 75,000 edible angiosperm species, of which maybe 7,000 are commonly consumed. Plants can be made into breads, pasta, cereals, juices, and jams, or raw materials like sugar, herbs, spices, and oils can be removed.

Sunflower, flaxseed, rapeseed (including canola oil), and sesame oils are extracted from oilseeds. Many plants and animals have coevolved in such a way that the fruit provides nourishment to the animal, which subsequently excretes the seeds some distance away, allowing for increased dissemination. Even seed predation can be mutually beneficial because some seeds survive digestion. Insects are the primary seed eaters, with ants being the sole true seed dispersers. Birds, despite being major dispersers, rarely eat seeds as a source of food and are distinguished by their strong beak that is employed to crack open the seed coat. Mammals eat a wider variety of seeds because their teeth can smash harder and larger seeds.

1.4 Diverse raw animal products

Animals are indirectly or directly utilized as sustenance. Meat, eggs, crustaceans, and dairy products such as milk and cheese are included. They are complete proteins suitable for human ingestion because they contain all of the essential amino acids required by the body. As such, they are an important source of protein. A steak, poultry breast, or pork chop weighing one ounce (110 grams) contains approximately 30 grams of protein. Protein is present in 7 grams per large egg. An approximately 15-gram (110 g) portion of cheese contains protein. Additionally, one cup of milk contains roughly eight grams of protein.

In addition to minerals, vitamins (including B12), lipids, and calories, animal products also contain essential vitamins (including iron, calcium, and magnesium). Animal-derived food items encompass mammary gland-produced milk, which is consumed or transformed into dairy products (cheese, butter, etc.) in numerous cultures. Consumed are eggs deposited by birds and other animals, while honey, a reduced form of floral nectar produced by bees, is a widely used sweetening agent in numerous cultures.

1.5 Food Taste

Five distinct flavors are typical of animals, including humans: sweet, sour, salty, bitter, and umami. The differentiation in flavor profiles serves a critical function in discerning nutritionally advantageous foods from those that potentially harbor detrimental contaminants. Throughout animal evolution, those flavors that impart the most energy have become the most palatable, whereas others have become unappealing.

However, it is worth noting that even humans are capable of developing a preference for substances that were initially unpleasant. Water, although vital for life, is tasteless. Sweetness is predominantly attributed to disaccharides, such as sucrose, a molecule formed by the combination of glucose and fructose, or simple sugars like fructose or glucose. Acidic substances, including the vinegar found in alcoholic beverages, produce sourness. Sour dishes consist of citrus fruits, particularly limes and lemons. The evolutionarily significant quality of sourness indicates that bacteria may have caused a product to become rancid. Sodium and potassium are examples of alkali metal ions that impart a salty flavor. Low to moderate amounts are present in nearly all foods for the purpose of augmenting flavor. A bitter taste is a disagreeable sensation distinguished by its sharp, pungent flavor. Certain fruit varieties, unsweetened dark chocolate, caffeine, and lemon rind are recognized for their bitterness. Umami, which is frequently defined as a flavor imparted to prepared meats and broths, serves as an indicator of protein content. Among the foods with a robust umami flavor are meat, dairy, and mushrooms.

1.6 The process of digestion

Composed of nutrient components, digestion breaks down food. Mechanical processes (chewing, peristalsis) and chemical processes (digestive enzymes and microorganisms) are required for proper digestion. Carnivores and herbivores have dissimilar digestive systems, as plant matter is considerably more difficult to metabolize. Carnivores possess mouths that are specifically engineered for shredding and biting, as opposed to herbivores' grinding mechanism. In contrast, herbivores possess slightly longer digestive tracts and more capacious intestines, which facilitate the process of cellulose digestion in plants. An omnivore is an animal that possesses the capacity to consume and endure on both plant and animal matter. Omnivores derive their energy and nutrients from plant and animal matter. In doing so, they metabolize the nutrients and energy absorbed from the sources they consume, which include carbohydrates, protein, lipids, and fiber. They frequently possess the capacity to integrate dietary sources including bacteria, algae, and fungi.

1.7 Carbohydrate

A carbohydrate is a type of biomolecule composed of carbon (C), hydrogen (H), and oxygen (O) atoms. Typically, the ratio of hydrogen to oxygen atoms is 2:1, similar to that of water. Therefore, the empirical formula for carbohydrates is Cm (H2O) n, where m and n may or may not be equal. It is important to note that in some cases, such as with CH_2O, hydrogen forms a covalent bond with carbon but not with oxygen. Nevertheless, certain carbohydrates such as uronic acids and deoxy-sugars like fucose do not strictly adhere to the stoichiometric criteria. Similarly, compounds like formaldehyde and acetic acid, despite meeting the definition, are not automatically categorized as carbs.

In the field of biochemistry, the term is frequently used as a synonym for saccharide, which derives from the Ancient Greek word σάκχαρον (sákkharon) meaning 'sugar'. This category encompasses sugars, starch, and cellulose. Saccharides are classified into four chemical categories: monosaccharides, disaccharides, oligosaccharides, and polysaccharides. Monosaccharides and disaccharides, which are the smallest carbohydrates with lower molecular weight, are often known as sugars. The scientific nomenclature of carbohydrates can be intricate, but the names of monosaccharides and disaccharides frequently have the suffix -ose. This suffix was derived from the word glucose, which originated from the Ancient Greek term γλεῦκος meaning 'wine' or 'must'. The -ose suffix is commonly used to denote various sugars, such as fructose (fruit sugar), sucrose (cane or beet sugar), ribose, lactose (milk sugar), and others.

Carbohydrates fulfill multiple functions in living beings. Polysaccharides function as both energy reserves (such as starch and glycogen) and structural elements (such as cellulose in plants and chitin in arthropods). Ribose, a monosaccharide with 5 carbon atoms, plays a crucial role as a constituent of coenzymes like as ATP, FAD, and NAD. Additionally, it serves as the structural foundation for RNA, the genetic material. Deoxyribose, which is closely associated, serves as a constituent of DNA. Saccharides and their derivatives encompass numerous vital biomolecules that fulfill crucial functions in the immune system, fertilization, pathogenesis prevention, blood clotting, and growth.

Carbohydrates play a fundamental role in nutrition and are present in a diverse range of both natural and processed foods. Starch is a complex carbohydrate that is found in high quantities in cereals (such as wheat, maize, and rice), potatoes, and processed foods made from cereal flour, such bread, pizza, or pasta. Sugars are mostly found in the human diet as table sugar (sucrose), which is obtained from sugarcane or sugar beets. Other common sugars include lactose, which is plentiful in milk, as well as glucose and fructose. Glucose and fructose are naturally present in honey, various fruits, and certain vegetables.

Drinks and various prepared dishes, such as jam, biscuits, and cakes, frequently incorporate table sugar, milk, or honey as ingredients. Cellulose, a polysaccharide present in the cell walls of all plants, constitutes a significant portion of indigestible dietary fiber. Cellulose and insoluble dietary fiber, while indigestible to humans, play a crucial role in promoting a healthy digestive system by aiding in regular bowel movements.

Additional polysaccharides included in dietary fiber consist of resistant starch and inulin. These substances serve as a source of nutrition for certain bacteria residing in the large intestine's microbiota. The bacteria metabolize these polysaccharides, resulting in the production of short-chain fatty acids.

1.8 Nutrient protein

Nutritionally, proteins are vital to human health. They can be used as fuel and are one among the components of biological tissue. Proteins have an energy density of 4 kcal (17 kJ) per gram, which is equal to that of carbohydrates; lipids have an energy density of 9 kcal (37 kJ) per gram. From a nutritional perspective, the composition of amino acids in protein is its most significant feature and distinguishing feature. Peptide bonds hold the amino acid chains in polymer chains that make up proteins. Proteins are broken down in the stomach by proteases and hydrochloric acid during human digestion, resulting in smaller polypeptide chains. This is necessary for the body to absorb the essential amino acids that are incapable of being biosynthesized.

Humans need to consume nine essential amino acids from their food in order to avoid protein-energy malnutrition and the death that follows. They are histidine, lysine, leucine, isoleucine, valine, threonine, tryptophan, and methionine. The question of whether there are eight or nine necessary amino acids has been debated. Because adults do not synthesize histidine, the general consensus seems to trend towards 9.

Humans may produce five different amino acids in their bodies. Alanine, aspartic acid, asparagine, glutamic acid, and serine are the five. Six amino acids are conditionally essential, meaning that their synthesis may be restricted in certain pathophysiological circumstances, such as newborn immaturity or acute catabolic distress. Arginine, cysteine, glycine, glutamine, proline, and tyrosine are the six. Grain, legumes, nuts, seeds, meats, dairy products, fish, eggs, edible insects, and seaweeds are dietary sources of protein.

1.8.1 The role of proteins in the human body

The human body need protein as one of its nutrients for growth and upkeep. Proteins are the most prevalent type of molecules in the body, next to water. Every single cell in the body is made mostly of protein, which serves as the structural foundation for all cells, including muscle. This also applies to skin, hair, and organs. Membranes also include proteins, including glycoproteins. They are utilized as building blocks for other molecules necessary for life, such as co-enzymes, hormones, immunological response, cellular repair, and nucleic acids, when they are broken down into amino acids. Protein is also required for the formation of blood cells.

1.8.2 Protein Sources

Protein can be found in many different foods. Plant-based foods provide for more than 60% of the global protein supply per person. Animal-derived foods make up over 70% of protein sources in North America. In many regions of the world, insects are a source of protein. Up to 50% of the protein in food is derived from insects in some parts of Africa. Over 2 billion individuals are thought to eat insects every day. Protein can be found in meat, dairy, eggs, soy, fish, whole grains, and cereals.

Food staples and cereal sources of protein that have a concentration of more than 7% include buckwheat, oats, rye, millet, maize (corn), rice, wheat, sorghum, amaranth, and quinoa, listed in no particular order. According to certain studies, game meat is a good source of protein. Legumes, nuts, seeds, grains, and some fruits and vegetables are plant sources of protein. Soybeans, lentils, kidney beans, white beans, mung beans, chickpeas, cowpeas, lima beans, pigeon peas, lupines, wing beans, almonds, Brazil nuts, cashews, pecans, walnuts, cotton seeds, pumpkin seeds, hemp seeds, sesame seeds, and sunflower seeds are just a few examples of plant foods that have higher protein content than 7%.

Using carbon dioxide from the atmosphere and electricity from solar panels, photovoltaic-driven microbial protein synthesis produces fuel for bacteria that are cultivated in bioreactor vats before being processed into dry protein powders. The method uses fertilizer, water, and land very efficiently. The US and Canadian Dietary Reference Intake guidelines state that in order to reduce the risk of deficiency, men and women aged 19 to 70 should consume 56 grams and 46 grams of protein daily, respectively. The 0.8 grams of protein per kilogram of body weight and the average body weights of 57 kg (126 pounds) and 70 kg (154 pounds), respectively, were used to compute these Recommended Dietary Allowances (RDAs). This approach, however, ignores the usage of protein for energy metabolism in favor of structural requirements. This prerequisite applies to the average inactive individual. The average protein intake in the US is higher than the RDA. The National Health and Nutrition Examination Survey (NHANES 2013–2014) found that men and women aged 20 over consumed 98.3 grams and 69.8 grams of protein on average per day, respectively.

1.8.3 People in action

Numerous studies have found that due to increased muscle mass and sweat losses, as well as the need for body repair and energy, athletes and active persons may need to consume higher amounts of protein (up to 0.8 g/kg). Although recommended daily consumption of protein is roughly 25%

of energy requirements, or 2 to 2.5 g/kg, for older adults, it varies from 1.2 to 1.4 g/kg for endurance exercisers to as high as 1.6-1.8 g/kg for strength exercisers and up to 2.0 g/kg/day for them. Nonetheless, there are still a lot of unanswered questions. Furthermore, some have proposed that in order to prevent the loss of lean muscle mass, athletes on low-calorie diets for weight loss should up their protein intake even higher, maybe to 1.8–2.0 g/kg.

1.8.4 Consumption in excess

An evaluation of dietary reference intakes for protein conducted in the United States and Canada came to the conclusion that there wasn't enough data to determine a tolerable upper intake level—that is, an upper limit on the amount of protein that may be ingested without risk. When the body requires more amino acids than it needs, the excess amino acids are taken up by the liver, which then deaminates them, turning the nitrogen into ammonia, which the liver then uses to produce urea through the urea cycle. Urea is eliminated by the kidneys. Glucose can be produced from other amino acid molecule components and utilized as fuel.

The body uses the "labile protein reserve" to make up for daily changes in protein consumption when food protein intake is sporadically high or low. This helps the body maintain equilibrium protein levels. There is no protein storage for later need, in contrast to body fat, which serves as a reserve for future calorie requirements. A diet high in protein may cause an increase in the excretion of calcium in the urine as a means of balancing the pH imbalance caused by the oxidation of sulfur amino acids. This could increase the likelihood that calcium in the renal circulatory system will produce kidney stones. Increased protein intake has no negative consequences on bone density, according to one meta-analysis. A different meta-analysis found no differences between diets high in animal or plant protein and a little drop in both systolic and diastolic blood pressure. In a meta-analysis, high protein diets were found to result in an extra 1.21 kg of weight loss over a 3-month period when compared to a baseline protein diet. Trials where protein consumption was just slightly increased showed stronger benefits of lowered body mass index and HDL cholesterol than trials where high protein intake was defined as 45% of total caloric intake. There were no negative effects on cardiovascular activity in those on short-term diets lasting six months or less.

There is disagreement over the long-term, high-protein diet's possible negative effects on healthy people, which has led to warnings against taking a high-protein diet to lose weight. Dietary Guidelines for Americans (DGA) 2015–2020 suggests that men and teenage boys improve their intake of fruits, vegetables, and other under-consumed foods. One way to achieve this is by consuming fewer items high in protein overall. There is no suggested upper limit on the consumption of red and processed meat in the 2015–2020 DGA report. The report highlights the importance of the nutrients found in red and processed meats, even as it acknowledges findings linking lesser intake of these meats to a lower risk of cardiovascular illnesses in adults. It is advised to monitor and maintain daily limits for sodium (< 2300 mg), saturated fats (less than 10% of daily calories), and added sugars (less than 10% of daily calories) that may increase due to consumption of specific meats and proteins rather than restricting intake of meats or protein. Although the 2015 DGA report suggests consuming fewer red and processed meats, the 2015–2020 DGA major recommendations suggest consuming a range of protein meals, including sources of protein that are both vegetarian and non-vegetarian.

1.9 Fat

Fat is often used in nutrition, biology, and chemistry to refer to any ester of fatty acids or a combination of such compounds, most commonly those found in living creatures or food. Triglycerides (triple esters of glycerol) are the major components of vegetable oils and fatty tissue in animals; alternatively, even more precisely, triglycerides that are solid or semisolid at room temperature, thereby excluding oils. The phrase can also be used more widely as a synonym for lipid, which is any biologically relevant material comprised of carbon, hydrogen, or oxygen that is insoluble in water but soluble in non-polar solvents. In this meaning, the term would cover several additional types of molecules, such as mono- and diglycerides, phospholipids (such as lecithin), sterols (such as cholesterol), waxes (such as beeswax), and free fatty acids, in addition to triglycerides.

Fats, along with carbohydrates and proteins, are one of the three major macronutrient groups in the human diet, and are the primary components of typical food products such as milk, butter, tallow, lard, salt pork, and cooking oils. They are a significant and dense source of nutritional energy for many animals, as well as crucial structural and metabolic functions in most living beings, including as energy storage, waterproofing, and thermal insulation. Except for a few essential fatty acids that must be included in the diet, the human body can generate the fat it needed from other food elements. Some flavor and fragrance compounds, as well as vitamins that are not water-soluble, are carried by dietary fats.

1.9.1 Biological significance

Fats function as both energy sources and storage for energy that the body does not require right away in humans and many animals. When fat is burned or digested, it produces around 9 food calories (37 kJ = 8.8 kcal). Fats also contain essential fatty acids, which are an important nutritional necessity. Vitamins A, D, E, and K are fat-soluble, which means they can only be digested, absorbed, and transported when they are combined with fat.

Fats are essential for maintaining healthy skin and hair, insulating body organs against shock, keeping the body temperature stable, and encouraging good cell function. Fat also acts as a protective barrier against a variety of ailments. When a specific molecule, whether chemical or biological, reaches dangerously high levels in the bloodstream, the body can effectively dilute—or at least maintain equilibrium with—the offending material by storing it in new fat tissue. This protects essential organs until the offending compounds may be digested or eliminated from the body by excretion, urine, accidental or purposeful bloodletting, sebum excretion, and hair growth.

1.9.2 Aspects of nutrition and health

Triglycerides are the most prevalent type of fat found in human diets and most living things. They are an ester of the triple alcohol glycerol $H(-CHOH-) 3H$ and three fatty acids. A triglyceride molecule is formed by a condensation reaction (specifically, esterification) between each of glycerol's -OH groups and the HO- part of the carboxyl group $HO(O=) C$ of each fatty acid, resulting in the formation of an ester bridge $O(O=) C$ and the elimination of a water molecule H_2O. Diglycerides and monoglycerides are less prevalent forms of lipids in which the esterification is limited to two or one of glycerol's -OH groups. Other alcohols, such as cetyl alcohol (which is prominent in spermaceti), may be used in place of glycerol. Phosphoric acid or a monoester thereof replaces one of the fatty acids in phospholipids.

The advantages and hazards of various amounts and types of dietary fats have been extensively researched and are still hotly debated topics. Fatty acids that are essential in human nutrition, there are two essential fatty acids (EFAs): alpha-Linolenic acid (an omega-3 fatty acid) and linoleic acid (an omega-6 fatty acid). Other lipids required by the adult body can be synthesized from these two.

1.9.3 Fats: Saturated vs. unsaturated

Different foods have varying amounts of fat with varying proportions of saturated and unsaturated fatty acids. Some animal products, such as beef and dairy products prepared with whole or reduced fat milk, such as yogurt, ice cream, cheese, and butter, are high in saturated fatty acids (and some are high in dietary cholesterol). Other animal items with primarily unsaturated fats include pig, poultry, eggs, and shellfish. Industrialized baked goods may also use fats with high unsaturated fat contents, particularly those containing partially hydrogenated oils, while processed foods deep-fried in hydrogenated oil have a high saturated fat content.

Plants and fish oil have a larger proportion of unsaturated acids, with the exceptions of coconut oil and palm kernel oil. Avocado, almonds, olive oils, and vegetable oils like canola are high in unsaturated fats. Many carefully conducted research have demonstrated that replacing saturated fats in the diet with cis unsaturated fats lowers the risk of cardiovascular disease (CVD), diabetes, and death.

Many medical organizations and public health departments, including the World Health Organization (WHO), were prompted by these findings to provide formal guidance. For these reasons, the United States Food and Drug Administration, for example, recommends consuming at least 10% (7% for high-risk groups) of total calories from saturated fat, with an average of 30% (or less) from all fat. The American Heart Association (AHA) also proposed a general 7% limit in 2006. The WHO/FAO report also suggested changing fats in order to minimize the quantity of myristic and palmitic acids in particular.

The so-called Mediterranean diet, which is popular in many Mediterranean Sea region countries, contains more total fat than Northern European diets, but the majority of it is in the form of unsaturated fatty acids (specifically, monounsaturated and omega-3) from olive oil and fish, vegetables, and certain meats like lamb, with little saturated fat consumption. According to a 2017 review, a Mediterranean-style diet may reduce the risk of cardiovascular disease, total cancer incidence, neurological illnesses, diabetes, and death rate. A 2018 review found that a Mediterranean-style diet may improve overall health by lowering the risk of noncommunicable diseases. It may help lower the social and economic consequences of dietary-related disorders. [We will have a detailed discussion on this later.]

1.10 Vitamin

Organic compounds known as vitamins, or a group of closely similar molecules known as vitamers, are necessary for an organism's correct metabolism when present in modest amounts. Essential nutrients must be received through diet since the body is unable to synthesize them in adequate amounts for survival. For instance, some species are able to synthesize vitamin C, but not others; in the former case, vitamin C is not regarded as a vitamin, but in the latter, it is.

Most vitamins are actually collections of related molecules called vitamers rather than single molecules. For instance, vitamin E is composed of eight different vitamins: four tocopherols and four tocotrienols. The three other categories of important nutrients—minerals, essential fatty acids, and essential amino acids—are not included in the word "vitamin."

Thirteen vitamins are listed by major health organizations:

• Provitamin A carotenoids, including all-trans beta-carotene, all-trans retinols, and all-trans retinyl esters

Vitamins B1 (thiamine), B2 (riboflavin), B3 (niacin), B5 (pantothenic acid), B6 (pyridoxine), B7 (biotin), B9 (folic acid and folates), B12 (cobalamins),

C (ascorbic acid and ascorbates),

and D (calciferols) should all be taken.

• Vitamin K (phylloquinones, menaquinones, and menadiones)

• Vitamin E (tocopherols and tocotrienols)

Choline is the fourteenth, according to certain sources.

Vitamins perform a variety of biochemical tasks. The proliferation and differentiation of cells and tissues is regulated by vitamin A. By controlling the metabolism of minerals in bones and other organs, vitamin D performs a role similar to that of a hormone. The vitamins in the B complex serve as precursors or cofactors for enzymes. Antioxidants include vitamins C and E.

Clinically severe sickness might potentially result from both excess and insufficient vitamin intake, while excess water-soluble vitamin intake is less likely to do so. Vitamin deficiency disorders have historically resulted from inadequate vitamin intake through diet. In order to prevent vitamin deficiencies in the general population, multivitamins and other vitamin supplements were mass produced and marketed in the 1950s. Food fortification, the process of adding certain vitamins to staple foods like milk or bread, is required by law in order to prevent vitamin deficiencies. Pregnancy-related folic acid supplementation guidelines decreased the risk of neural tube abnormalities in unborn children.

1.10.1 Sources of Intake

Most vitamins are acquired through the diet, but some can be obtained in other ways. For instance, certain types of vitamin K and biotin are produced by gut flora microorganisms, and skin cells can synthesize one type of vitamin D when they are exposed to specific UV light wavelengths found in sunlight. Certain vitamins can be made by humans from precursors they eat; for instance, beta carotene is used to make vitamin A, while tryptophan is used to make niacin. Certain species are able to manufacture vitamin C, whereas others cannot. The only vitamin or nutrient that cannot be obtained from plants is vitamin B12. The Food Fortification Initiative maintains a list of nations with folic acid, niacin, vitamin A, and vitamins B1, B2, and B12 required fortification programs.

1.11 Salt - that is edible

Salt is vital for human and animal health, and it is one of the five basic taste senses. Salt is utilized in a variety of cuisines, and it is frequently present in salt shakers on diners' dining tables for personal use on food. Many processed foods contain salt as an ingredient. Table salt is a refined salt that contains 97-99 percent sodium chloride. To make it free-flowing, anticaking chemicals such as sodium aluminosilicate or magnesium carbonate are usually used. Iodized salt (potassium iodide) is commonly available. Some individuals add a desiccant in their salt shakers, such as a few grains of uncooked rice or a saltine cracker, to absorb extra moisture and help break up salt clumps that may form.

1.11.1 Table salt with added nutrients

Some table salt supplied for human consumption has chemicals that treat a number of health issues, particularly in developing countries. The identities and amounts of additives vary by country. Iodine is an essential micronutrient for humans, and a lack of it can result in decreased thyroxine production (hypothyroidism) and thyroid gland hypertrophy (endemic goitre) in adults or cretinism in children. Iodized salt, which consists of table salt mixed with a trace amount of potassium iodide, sodium iodide, or sodium iodate, has been used to treat these conditions since 1924. To stabilize the iodine, a small amount of dextrose may be added. Iodine deficiency affects around two billion people globally and is the greatest preventable cause of intellectual disability. Iodized table salt has greatly reduced iodine deficient illnesses in nations where it is utilized.

The amount of iodine and the type of iodine compound that is added to salt varies. The Food and Drug Administration (FDA) recommends 150 micrograms of iodine per day for both men and women in the United States. Iodized salt in the United States contains 46-77 ppm (parts per million), however in the United Kingdom, the recommended iodine concentration of iodized salt is 10-22 ppm.

"Doubly fortified salt" contains both iodide and iron salts. The latter addresses iron deficiency anaemia, which affects the mental development of an estimated 40% of infants in underdeveloped countries. Ferrous fumarate is a common iron source. Folic acid (vitamin B9), which gives table salt its yellow color, is another ingredient that is very helpful for pregnant women. Folic acid aids in the prevention of neural tube abnormalities and anaemia, both of which affect young mothers, particularly in underdeveloped nations.

A lack of fluoride in the diet causes a significant rise in the incidence of dental caries. Fluoride salts can be added to table salt to reduce tooth decay, particularly in areas where fluoridated toothpaste and water are not available.

1.11.2 Other types

Unrefined sea salt contains trace amounts of algal products, salt-resistant microorganisms, and sediment particles, as well as magnesium and calcium halides and sulfates. The calcium and magnesium salts impart a somewhat bitter aftertaste and make unrefined sea salt hygroscopic (it progressively collects moisture from the air if stored exposed). Algal products give off a moderately "fishy" or "sea-air" odor, the latter due to organobromine chemicals. The salt has a drab grey color due to sediments, the percentage of which varies depending on the source. Because taste and scent components are typically discernible by humans in minute concentrations, when sprinkled on top of food, sea salt may have a more nuanced flavor than pure sodium chloride. However, when salt is added during cooking, these flavors are likely to be overpowered by those of the food ingredients. According to scientific investigations, raw sea and rock salts do not contain enough iodine salts to prevent iodine deficient disorders.

Kosher salt, also known as kitchen salt, contains larger grains than table salt and is used in cooking. When coupled with oil, it can be used for brining, bread or pretzel manufacturing, and as a scouring agent.

1.11.3 Food containing salt

Most meals include salt, however it is present in very minute amounts in naturally occurring foods such as meats, vegetables, and fruit. It is frequently added to processed foods (such as canned goods, particularly salted foods, pickled foods, and snack foods or other convenience foods), where it serves as a preservative as well as a seasoning. Dairy salt is used in the production of butter and cheese. Salt enhances the flavor of other foods by decreasing their bitterness, making them more pleasant and substantially sweeter.

Prior to the invention of electrically driven refrigeration, one of the primary techniques of food preservation was salting. Thus, herring has 67 mg of sodium per 100 g, whereas kipper, the preserved variety, has 990 mg. Similarly, pork contains 63 mg per 100 g, whereas bacon contains 1,480 mg, and potatoes contain 7 mg, but potato crisps carry 800 mg per 100 g. Salt is also widely used in cuisine as a seasoning, as well as in cooking techniques like as salt crusts and brining. Apart from the direct usage of sodium chloride, the main sources of salt in the Western diet include bread and cereal items, meat products, and milk and dairy products.

Salt is not traditionally used as a condiment in many East Asian cultures. Condiments like soy sauce, fish sauce, and oyster sauce, on the other hand, have a high sodium concentration and serve a comparable function to table salt in western cultures. They are more commonly used in cooking than as table condiments.

1.11.4 Sodium intake and health

Because table salt contains just under 40% sodium by weight, a 6 g serving (1 teaspoon) contains around 2,400 mg of sodium. Sodium performs an important function in the human body: as an electrolyte, it aids nerve and muscle activity, and it is one of the factors involved in the osmotic regulation of water content in body organs (fluid balance). The majority of sodium in the Western diet comes from salt. Many Western countries consume roughly 10 g of salt per day, which is greater than in many Eastern European and Asian countries. The high salt content of many processed foods has a significant impact on the total amount consumed. In the United States, 75% of the sodium consumed comes from processed and restaurant foods, 11% from cooking and table use, and the remainder from naturally occurring in foods.

Because consuming too much sodium raises the risk of cardiovascular disease, health organizations generally advise people to limit their salt intake. High sodium consumption is linked to an increased risk of stroke, overall cardiovascular disease, and kidney disease. A 1,000 mg reduction in sodium intake per day may lower cardiovascular risk by roughly 30%. A decrease in sodium intake from typical high levels lowers blood pressure in adults and children who do not have an acute illness. In persons with hypertension, a low sodium diet results in a larger improvement in blood pressure.

The World Health Organization recommends that individuals take no more than 2,000 mg of sodium per day (the amount found in 5 g of salt). According to US guidelines, those with hypertension, African Americans, and middle-aged and older adults should limit their sodium consumption to no more than 1,500 mg per day and reach the potassium target of 4,700 mg/day through a nutritious diet of fruits and vegetables.

While developed countries recommend limiting sodium intake to less than 2,300 mg per day, one review suggested limiting sodium intake to at least 1,200 mg (contained in 3 g of salt) per day, as the greater the reduction in salt intake, the greater the fall in systolic blood pressure for all age groups and ethnicities. Another assessment concluded that there is inadequate data to decide if lowering sodium consumption to less than 2,300 mg per day is beneficial or detrimental.

Evidence suggests that the association between salt and cardiovascular disease is more convoluted. "Mortality caused by levels of salt the association between sodium consumption and cardiovascular disease or mortality is U-shaped, with increased risk at both high and low sodium intake." The findings revealed that those with hypertension were more likely to die as a result of excessive salt consumption. Regardless of blood pressure, the levels of increased mortality among those with restricted salt intake appeared to be identical. This research suggests that, while those with hypertension should focus primarily on lowering sodium to suggested levels, all groups should strive to maintain a healthy sodium intake of 4 to 5 grams (equal to 10-13 g salt) per day.

Diets high in salt are one of the world's two most major dietary concerns for impairment.

2.0: Female weight vs Male weight - who gets the stigma?

Is weight gain an inevitable outcome for every individual? Is weight gain a hereditary feature or mainly due to lifestyle? We will explore the conspicuous as well as mysterious ways weight creep up into our mortal structure.

Although our whole discussion is centered around women, shedding light on the male counterparts - as well - would help us appreciate the extent of the problem in a more subtle way. Hence, this brief exploration delves into the factors impacting male aging issue and some tips to avert many of the detrimental consequences of age-related development.

2.1 The Changing Male Form

If you are a male, you have watched your physique evolve throughout the years.

Perhaps you've gained some weight or found that your hairline has shifted since you were younger. Knowing how a man's body changes as he matures can help him make informed decisions about his health and well-being at any stage of his life.

As you proceed on your path to health, keep in mind these shifts:

Fat

From the time they hit their 30s, most men continue to put on weight consistently until they reach their 55s. Men are more likely to develop heart disease and other health problems if they are overweight and keep that weight on throughout life. Measuring your waist circumference is a quick and easy approach to see if you're carrying too much weight. Aim for a healthier size if it measures more than 40 inches. The good news is that your belly fat is the first to disappear when you start losing weight as a guy.

Muscle

As your male hormones begin to diminish around middle age, you'll gradually lose muscular mass. Maintaining a regular strength training regimen as you age is beneficial since it can prevent further muscle and bone loss, as well as increase testosterone levels. Aim for two weekly strength-training sessions separated by at least one day of rest for the muscles being worked (you can engage in other forms of exercise, such as cardio, or strength-train different muscles on the rest days). Work out your major muscle groups with eight to ten sets of various exercises.

Heart

Even though heart disease is uncommon in men in their thirties and forties, risk factors might emerge suddenly. By the time males reach the age of 50 to 64, hypertension affects more than half of them. The elasticity of the arteries and veins decreases with age, even in a healthy person, which increases the risk of hypertension. It's never too early (or too late) to follow a preventive lifestyle, which includes frequent screening. Screenings for high blood pressure and cholesterol are recommended annually for healthy males and every five years for those with risk factors. Once you reach 45, discuss taking an aspirin daily with your doctor to reduce your risk of a heart attack.

Prostate

As you become older, this normally little organ expands. If your urethra or bladder is being compressed, you may feel the urge to urinate frequently or have involuntary urination. However, the same heart-healthy habits that reduce the risk of cardiovascular disease also reduce the chance of prostate cancer as you become older. Screening should begin with an annual manual prostate exam beginning at age 40; the use of the prostate-specific antigen (PSA) test is controversial and should be discussed with your doctor.

Penis

Although many men maintain normal sexual function long into old age, other men notice a decline in erection frequency and in their ability to have numerous sexual encounters. Libido, or sexual desire, can also decrease with age. Cardiovascular disease, which can reduce blood flow to the penis, is the most common cause of erectile dysfunction.

Skin

Age-related changes to the skin include a diminished ability to heal wounds and a heightened sensitivity to the cold. Even if you haven't given it much thought before, it's in your best interest to start doing so now. Avoid tanning beds, always apply a sunscreen with UVA and UVB protection, keep your skin hydrated, and take care of any cuts or scratches right away. Solar keratosis, which causes crusty, rough spots, is more common beyond the age of 45. Since this is a precursor to cancer, you should discuss with your doctor whether or not a skin cancer screening might be beneficial to you. See a dermatologist if you notice any unusual changes to your skin.

Hair

Male pattern baldness affects roughly 50% of males. Some men with a hereditary predisposition to hair loss may notice it as early as their college years, but most people who experience thinning do so sometime between the ages of 30 and 40. The typical area to start thinning out is the crown of the head, giving rise to the dreaded "bald spot." Although thinning hair isn't necessarily dangerous, men who experience premature balding may be at a higher risk for cardiovascular disease and prostate cancer. That just means you have more reason to adopt the kind of preventative lifestyle that every man (and woman) should aim for.

2.2 Now turning to women:

Does the particular age boundary over 50 a blessing in the society for their wealth of experience or a source of indignation for the younger age group? Since every living entity - the human one - has to go through this age bracket if they can breathe well into their forties, will they consider 50 or more as just another year in the calendar or a handwriting on the wall?

How your weight changes as you get older

For how long does your weight stay the same? As women age, one change that is easy to see is that their body fat percentage goes up. People often lose muscle strength as they age, which makes their bodies feel weaker than they did when they were younger. Women may also get wrinkles because their skin is less flexible and strong, or their hair may thin and turn gray. Men usually stop adding body fat around age 55, but women tend to keep gaining weight until they are 65. This is because as people get older, their metabolism slows down, making it harder to keep the weight off or lose it. After menopause, this extra weight moves from the hips and legs to the middle.

2.3 Body Parts That Change:
Bones and muscles

We lose a lot of muscle as we age, which makes us weaker and less able to keep up with activities for long periods of time. Some loss is normal with getting older, but it's also caused by things like less exercise, not getting enough nutrients, and long-term illnesses. As we get older, the structures that lubricate and cushion our joints change. This makes it harder for our bodies to heal from repeated stress and makes our joints feel stiffer. As the tissues in our joints wear away, we may get arthritis.

From youth to about age 30, bone density goes up, especially if you work out regularly and eat a lot of calcium and vitamin D. Around age 35, bone loss starts slowly because hormone levels change. During and after menopause, women lose an average of 0.5% to 1.5% of their body weight each year. It can be as high as 3 to 5 percent per year for people who lose bone mass quickly. Your risk of breaking a bone goes up as your bones get smaller and more porous, and you may also get shorter. Loss of height is caused by things like squished discs, changes in the legs and feet, and smaller joint areas. From age 65 on, the National Osteoporosis Foundation says that women should get a bone density test. Women are told to get it before they turn 50 because by age 65, women already have a 50% chance of getting a fragility fracture in their lives.

How Hearts of Women Change as They Get Older

Heart disease is much less likely to happen to women who eat well, work out regularly, and don't smoke. But heart disease rates are two to three times higher in women who are menopausal than in women of the same age who are not menopausal. Heart attacks become more common about ten years after menopause, according to studies. They are the main cause of death in older women.

Aging and Breasts

When a woman goes through events in her life, like puberty and birth, her breasts change. When a woman goes through menopause, her estrogen levels drop. This makes her breasts less big and elastic, which is called "sagging."

The National Cancer Institute says that women's risk of getting breast cancer also goes up as they age. Women have an 8% chance of getting breast cancer: The chance of getting breast cancer in the next ten years for a woman 30 years old is just under 0.5%. The chance for a woman 60 years old is just above 3.5%, or 1 in 28.

How Your Pelvic and Reproductive Health Has Changed

As people age, many of them find it harder and harder to hold their pee. It happens to about 1 in 10 people over 65. During menopause, dry vaginal tissue may make sex more painful and make urinary tract infections more likely. Moisturizers and lubricants can help with sexual pain and dryness. (Some doctors may recommend low-dose vaginal estrogen to treat chronic UTIs caused by low estrogen levels. This will raise hormone levels and good bacteria levels. Making changes to your lifestyle, like having more water to get rid of bacteria that are bad for your urinary tract, might help. If it's long-lasting and happens often, doctors will probably give you medicines.)

Some women feel less young, beautiful, and physically attractive during menopause because of the changes that happen. Strong muscles and ligaments that support your pelvic floor are important for your sexual, reproductive, and urine health. Pelvic organ prolapses (where the pelvic organs slip out of place) and urine incontinence can happen after giving birth, having a hysterectomy, or going through menopause.

The collagen fibers in the top layer of your skin may get rougher and less organized after age 50. This makes your skin less flexible, which makes lines stand out more. It also makes less natural oil, which makes your skin feel dry and tight. Melanocytes that make pigments drop, which makes sun-related skin cancers more likely.

How Hair Adapts to Age

Your hair thins out and grows more slowly as you get older. If you've been finding more hairs in your brush, don't worry.

About 80% of people lose some hair over time, especially after age 50. Most women start graying their hair in their 30s, but some women get it younger if their genes make it so. Like in the skin, hair turns gray when melanocytes are lost from hair roots. The number of hair follicles on the head and hair growth rates in other parts of the body both slow down as people age. We don't want hair to grow in places we don't want it to, like on our faces.

Immune System Changes

As soon as reaching the age mark of 50, the immune system can progressively weaken to allow invasion of viruses or external intimidations capable of causing infections or any other ailment. In addition, the quantity of cells combating in our body will also encounter diminution and we are ought to fall prey to diseases while having a go with a virus, bacteria or pathogen. Due to all this, anyone is susceptible to be down with the flu, pneumonia, or even tetanus.

Brain Health

Treading into 50 will be not like the one in our 25 in terms of brain function.

There might be a dipping of slightly about age 55, dwelling on that notion will not be a good idea.

According to specialists, perception of yourself having a slower cerebral function with the progression of age may lead to such reality.

Mental Health

Approximately 95% of individuals who have reached 50 or gone beyond may express their satisfaction or even ecstasy with their living status. Nevertheless, in women, the hormone change due to menopause can trigger fluctuations in temperament. If we add illness and substantial amount of alcohol consumption. The likelihood of depression can spike easily. A humble approach for the enhancement temper: Sitting less often and moving frequently. Our odds of mental health problems escalate if we remain seated above 7 hours a day or go for workout.

Hearing

Equal to 40% of individuals over 50 experience auditory compromise. Besides aging naturally, our genetic composition can have their role, and some health difficulties -- such as diabetes, heart problems, and high blood pressure -- can distress our hearing ability in the course of time.

In case of having complications, it is advisable to consult a physician for the hearing impairment detection. Individuals unable to hear properly have greater probability to be dissociated from their near ones, eventually leading to depression.

3.0:   Graceful Ageing - myth or reality?

How do we perceive aging? Is it the scariest notion for most of the individuals? Does culture have any bearing on the perception? Is aging consistent with time or condition? We need to understand these because we have to relate the aging concept with weight theories.

In a culture that values being young and thin, the normal changes that come with getting older are often not accepted. Some women turn to makeup and plastic surgery to try to stop time from passing them by. Others worry too much about their weight and start to dislike their bodies. This can hurt your self-esteem and make you want to stay away from people. Learning about how your body naturally ages can help, though. It's true that as we age, our bodies slowly lose the ability to do things and heal themselves. Health issues and medicines can speed up these changes. You can change how you take care of your health, though, to keep your mind and body in good shape for as long as possible. It is important to take care of your body, mind, and heart at all times in your life.

Wisdom, empathy, and experience are acquired via life's experiences. Many women feel more appreciative of each day that goes by, more self-assured in their choices, and more equipped to allocate their time when they reach 50 years of age and beyond. However, doctors also believe that aging begins to take its toll on physical health around age 50, leading to sometimes unanticipated changes.

Menopause's shifting hormone levels make aging more severe for women's bodies, according to Kathryn Rexrode, M.D., Harvard Medical School professor of medicine and head of the women's health division at Brigham and Women's Hospital. In the United States, the average age of menopause is 51. Menopause officially begins one year following a woman's last menstrual cycle. According to Rexrode, "for women, 50 is an age that is an inflection point, when biological aging is catching up." "Women ask, 'What's happening to my body? It was acting one way before, but it's acting differently now." The good news is that you have a number of options for how to react to those modifications. According to Rexrode, "there are many things we can do to keep our bodies healthy and vibrant as we age, but yes, there are certain changes in our bodies that we need to accept."

Women over fifty sometimes ask their doctors, "Why am I gaining weight when I haven't changed my diet or exercise routine?" Why is the metabolism of women over 50 slower? Our metabolism slows down as we get older because we lose lean muscle mass. Additionally, we often become less active and burn less calories, which contributes to weight gain.

Is this a typical issue? Indeed, even from extremely fit patients. Women typically notice the slow, steady weight gain around the age of 40 to 50. They could have lost weight by giving up a snack in the past. Now, however, the scale remains stationary when they do that. Why does it seem that males can lose weight more easily now than women can? Men lose muscle and their metabolism slows down with age. However, they do not experience the same hormonal fluctuations as women do. The absence of estrogen during menopause causes fat to migrate to the middle of the body. The risk of heart disease, stroke, and type 2 diabetes is raised by this belly fat.

3.1 Disorders of eating in midlife

Bulimia, anorexia, and binge eating do not only affect youthful people. Decades-long extreme dietary behaviors are motivated by what?

How does one manifest an eating disorder? A youthful, waiflike woman strutting down a catwalk while protruding bones beneath her clothing is a thought that is likely to occur to one. Her older sisters, however, are not impervious to anorexia, bulimia, or compulsive eating. Contrary to conventional belief, a greater proportion of women in their mid-life and beyond embark on perilous weight-control journeys.

It is common knowledge that the majority of us have dieted at some point, with some of us doing so frequently. However, Harvard experts say that as we age, women may encounter unique stressors that increase their risk of developing eating disorders. Specifically, the rigors of calorie restriction or binge-purge cycles can exacerbate health effects in the elderly.

One in every five women has experienced an eating disorder by the time they reach the age of 40, which is twice the percentage of women diagnosed at age 21 (JAMA Network Open, 2019). Dr. Holly Peek, associate medical director of the Klarman Eating Disorders Center at McLean Hospital, which is affiliated with Harvard, explains that many cases are probably the resurgence of a pattern that may have escaped detection in previous years.

"Many women with eating disorders in midlife have had the problem for most of their lives," according to Dr. Peek. "And a lot are going through major life transitions starting around age 40 that are all different from those of a teenage or young woman."

Additionally, disordered eating that erroneously straddles the boundary between normal and problematic is far more prevalent than officially diagnosed eating disorders. It may manifest as chronic starvation, yo-yo dieting, or excessive exercise until midlife. "Adolescents may become excessively preoccupied with their image as gym rats who adhere to a strict diet, and menopause-induced changes in their bodies cause them to lose sight of the truth," explains Dr. Peek. "They might not even perceive it as a problem." "Everything becomes extremely complicated."

3.2 Twenty-year-old risk factors

Although there exists a wide range of eating disorders, only three are prevalent: anorexia nervosa, which is distinguished by its extreme restriction of food intake; binge eating disorder, which involves binge eating until fullness is experienced; and bulimia nervosa, which entails gorging followed by purging via regurgitation or laxative use.

Anorexia becomes less prevalent after the age of 26, whereas bulimia prevalence does not peak until the age of 47, according to a study published in the International Journal of Eating Disorders in November 2017. Binge eating disorder, which is the most prevalent eating disorder among adults overall, may persist as an issue for women in their seventies.

Over the decades, what has sustained such a pathological preoccupation with food and weight? Midlife and elder women may be reentering the dating scene following a divorce or widowhood, or they may be attempting to maintain a competitive edge in the workplace, where thinness is often associated with youth. Additionally, the shock of a deserted nest may inspire body-redefining endeavors.

"The significance of body image appears to be a crucial factor in whether or not women develop or return to an eating disorder," according to Harvard University Health Services primary care physician Dr. Bettina Bentley. "With aging, many women are also disturbed by the lack of control over the ways their body is changing."

In fact, estrogen fluctuations associated with the transition to menopause can increase the risk of developing an eating disorder. "We know that estrogen plays a role in developing an eating disorder on both ends of the age spectrum, but in terms of why, the jury is still out," according to Dr. Peek. "Women during menopause are more likely to gain weight, and you may feel your body is working against you."

3.3 Diverse health consequences

Irrespective of external appearance, eating disorders can have detrimental effects on the body. Women with eating disorders frequently suffer from nutrient deficiencies, especially in iron, vitamin B12, calcium, and vitamin D, according to Margaret Schrier, chief of nutrition at Harvard University Health Services and a registered dietitian. "Supplements can help with deficiencies and are usually well tolerated by patients," Schrier asserts. It is recommended to take them with food, as absorption may be diminished when taken on an empty stomach.

Malnutrition, extreme weight loss, and purging can also result in the following complications:

Loss of bone mass.

Dr. Bentley states that the risk of bone fracture is seven times greater in individuals with anorexia compared to the general population. Although bone density testing is not typically advised for women in their fifties, she prescribes it for those whom she suspects may be suffering from an eating disorder or have experienced bone fractures.

Heart complications.

Disrupted electrolyte balance resulting from a dietary disorder may contribute to tachycardia. Additionally, midlife women are more likely to be prescribed medications to treat chronic conditions, which can heighten this risk. "It's more of a recipe for a medical emergency, because your body just isn't as resilient as when you were 16," according to Dr. Peek.

Lung disorders.

Muscles of the chest deteriorate with time, particularly in individuals who compel themselves to vomit repeatedly. This increases the risk of pneumonia.

Intestinal disorders.

Constipation, diarrhea, reflux, bloating, nausea, vomiting, or constipation may be associated with an eating disorder rather than age-related symptoms.

Illness with diabetes.

Binge eaters have significantly higher rates of diabetes, according to Dr. Bentley, which is likely fueled by the frequent blood sugar spikes that occur after binge eating.

Skin deterioration.

Long-term anorexics frequently develop severe facial wrinkling and ineffective wound healing, according to Dr. Bentley. This is likely indicative of a chronic nutritional deficiency.

Although eating disorders are the leading cause of death among psychiatric illnesses, only 27% of those afflicted attempt to seek professional assistance. An interdisciplinary health team, comprising a therapist and dietitian, can assist individuals in achieving optimal physical and mental health. If you suspect that you may be suffering from an eating disorder, do not hesitate to candidly discuss the matter with your physician. Without prejudice, she is trained to evaluate and treat eating disorders as she would any other medical condition.

3.4 Grace of Aging

With all the discussion at our disposal, now some wise words: Remember that the passing of time has many benefits as you go through these and other changes. Some things you may enjoy as you age are not having to worry about birth control and having kids who are grown up and living on their own. You might notice a change in how you feel, like not having to please other people as much. You might also find that now is a good time to get back in touch with your true loves and joys. In general, older people are more responsible, friendly, and content than people in their mid-40s.

3.5 More advice on how to age well

Stay away from processed and sugary foods because they make diseases like Alzheimer's and diabetes worse. Drinking too much booze can lead to oxidative stress, which speeds up the aging process. Get enough rest and deal with your stress. Grow your relationships with family and friends. The most important thing is to stay busy. Older people who stay active often act like they are younger.

3.6 Age Related Problems:

Diagnosis of Problem: Should you test or not?

Teresa Fung, an adjunct professor of nutrition at the Harvard T.H. Chan School of Public Health, says that some of us aren't getting enough nutrients unless we consciously skip whole food groups or drastically cut back on our food intake. "We're a country of excess consumption," she says. Not having enough food to eat is a big problem in the United States, but if you eat a lot of different kinds of food at different times each day, you probably aren't lacking in calories or nutrients.

Still, because of age, hormone changes, or other things, women can certainly not get enough of a few vitamins and minerals. These are the nutrients that people are most likely to not get enough of.

Symptoms, or the lack of them, are not always a sign that you may not be getting enough nutrients. Blake says that most flaws are minor and don't show up right away. It's also not something you can figure out on your own.

"The term 'deficiency' is really a medical term," Fung says. "If you put your food into an app that tells you what nutrients it contains, it still won't tell you if you are deficient." That needs to be checked by a doctor."

Also, our bodies store small amounts of extra vitamins and minerals that would last us for a few weeks if we didn't eat well. This means that our levels would have to be very low before a problem shows up. For example, a lack of vitamin D might only show up when a bone breaks.

Fung says that a blood test is not a good way to figure out calcium amounts. Usually, though, blood tests can tell you if you're not getting enough of important nutrients like vitamin D, iron, or B12. There's "no need to test for every deficiency under the sun," but Fung says you should ask your doctor if she thinks your risk factors mean you should take a closer look. "If you're concerned or even curious, it's absolutely worth a conversation with your doctor," states Blake.

3.7: Why do you need a multivitamin?

Big boxes, bright colors, and even candies that look like candy: Multivitamins are easy to take and taste good. It might feel like nutrition insurance to take a pill or drink a special mixture every day that has a mix of vitamins, minerals, and other nutrients.

Teresa Fung, an associate professor of nutrition at the Harvard T.H. Chan School of Public Health, says there's no need if you're healthy in general and eat a variety of foods. "A vitamin pill does not contain all the beneficial stuff in food," Fung states. "It's not a shortcut."

But the following things make it more likely that someone will gain from multivitamins:

Age.

As people age, they may have trouble eating and swallowing or lose the desire to eat enough.

Giving birth.

Since many pregnancies happen without planning to, women of childbearing age should think about taking a daily multivitamin with the B vitamin folate, which is also known as folic acid. If taken early in pregnancy, this vitamin can lower the chance of brain and spinal cord defects in the developing embryo.

Problems with digestion.

Some health problems, like celiac disease, ulcerative colitis, and cystic fibrosis, can make eating hard. So can gastric bypass surgery, which cuts out parts of the digestive system to help people lose weight.

Certain medicines.

 People who take proton-pump inhibitors for heartburn and acid reflux may not be able to receive vitamin B12 properly. Some medicines for Parkinson's disease can also stop your body from absorbing B vitamins. Also, diuretics, which are used to lower blood pressure, can use up your magnesium, potassium, and calcium stores.

Autoimmune diseases may be avoided with vitamin D and fish oil.

There are more than 24 million people in the United States who have autoimmune diseases like rheumatoid arthritis, eczema, or thyroid disease. But so far, scientists haven't found any possible ways to stop these painful conditions, which mostly affect women.

Now, though, a study from Harvard suggests that people over 50 may be able to avoid getting autoimmune diseases by taking vitamin D and fish oil supplements. There are more than 80 of these diseases that happen when the immune system attacks healthy cells, tissues, or organs by accident. Their signs are different, but they may include pain, tiredness, skin issues, and other long-term issues.

She led the main Vitamin D and Omega-3 Trial (VITAL) and co-wrote the new report, which came out in The BMJ on January 26, 2022. "We were surprised that a signal for a benefit could emerge for such a broad and varied group of diseases," says Dr. JoAnn Manson, chief of the Division of Preventive Medicine at Harvard-affiliated Brigham and Women's Hospital. "Because there are no known ways to prevent autoimmune diseases — whether lifestyle, diet, or medications — these results were exciting."

3.7.1 Effects on fighting inflammation

How do you think vitamin D and fish oil might help fight inflammatory disease? Because they can control the immune system and reduce inflammation, which is what causes autoimmune diseases, researchers thought that the pair might be able to avoid them. That's because women are at least four times more likely than men to be diagnosed with an autoimmune disease. The results are important for women. But, according to Dr. Manson, it's too early to say that everyone should take vitamin D or fish oil pills to try to avoid getting autoimmune diseases. Also, these vitamins should be studied more in people who are more likely to get autoimmune diseases and in younger adults, since these diseases tend to start before, they turn 30.

"But those with a strong family history, or who have been told they may have early signs of an autoimmune disorder, may want to talk with their health care providers about whether to begin taking these supplements," explains Dr. Manson.

3.8 How can a dietary disorder be identified?

A person who experiences extreme weight loss has an eating disorder. However, what other methods could you employ to identify this condition in yourself or others?

Consider the following:

• significant variations in body weight, irrespective of whether it is increasing or decreasing;

• fixation on weight, calories, body shape, and body image;

• aversion to specific food items or food categories (e.g., carbohydrates or sugar);

• excessive physical activity;

• meal skipping or consumption of minute portions during scheduled meals;

• food rituals, including excessive chewing or preventing different foods on a plate from touching;

• indications of purging behaviors, including frequent trips to the restroom and sounds of vomiting;

"It is a sign to seek help whenever these thoughts and behaviors take over your life," advises Dr. Holly Peek, associate medical director of McLean Hospital's Klarman Eating Disorders Center.

4.0: Diving deep into the weight pool - the weight gain theories

Our most important concept to delve into will be this one. All the buildup prior was for this chapter which would be elaborating all the hypotheses and theories till date regarding weight gain and loss issues. It is obvious that without understanding the nuances of this most complex reality, we would be at the mercy of wild guesses rather than making judicious decisions of our own.

Hormonal changes, such as lower estrogen and testosterone levels, occur as we age. These alterations can have an impact on how our bodies store fat, particularly in the abdominal area. This abdominal fat might be tough to shed, making weight reduction more difficult as we get older.

Excess sugar consumption contributes significantly to the buildup of abdominal fat. Consuming a lot of sugar produces an increase in insulin levels. Insulin is a hormone that controls blood sugar levels; however, if levels remain chronically raised owing to excessive sugar consumption, it can develop to insulin resistance.

Insulin resistance develops when the cells of the body become less sensitive to the actions of insulin. This condition can cause weight gain and make losing weight even more difficult. When the body develops insulin resistance, it has trouble processing glucose for energy properly, leading in greater blood sugar levels and increased fat accumulation, particularly in the abdomen.

Snacking late at night can have a detrimental impact on appetite, hormones, metabolism, and body fat distribution. Take a look at the following:

1.   Increased hunger and changes in appetite-controlling hormones:

Late-night eating can throw off the natural circadian cycle of appetite-regulating hormones like ghrelin and leptin. This disturbance can lead to increased hunger and an increased proclivity to overeat, making it more difficult to stick to a sensible eating plan.

2.   Reduced calorie burning:

According to a study published in Cell Metabolism, eating late at night may lower the quantity of calories expended throughout the day when compared to eating earlier in the day. This is related to the body's normal metabolic swings as well as lower activity levels at night.

3.   Fat storage in the belly:

Late-night eating has been linked to an increased risk of fat storage in the abdomen. This form of fat, called visceral fat, has been associated to an elevated risk of a variety of health problems, including cardiovascular disease and type 2 diabetes.

Certain drugs, particularly those intended to treat illnesses that are exacerbated by excess weight, such as heart disease and type 2 diabetes, can promote weight gain. According to research published in Obesity, more than 20% of individuals in the United States use at least one weight-gaining medicine. Beta-blockers and diabetic medicines such as insulin and sulfonylureas are among the most commonly connected with weight gain.

Hormones, steroids, and some antidepressants, in addition to these drugs, can lead to weight gain. The longer these drugs are used, the more massive and stubborn fat cells the body may store. Individuals using these drugs may find it more difficult to lose weight as a result of this.

Adequate sleep is essential for keeping a healthy weight. Sleep deprivation is regularly linked to weight growth, according to research. Research published in BMJ Open Sport & Exercise Medicine found that sleep-deprived individuals not only consumed more food the next day, but also preferred high-calorie alternatives.

Sleep deprivation can interfere with the body's ability to regulate hunger hormones like ghrelin, which stimulates appetite, and leptin, which suppresses hunger. When you don't get enough sleep, your ghrelin levels rise, causing you to eat more, while your leptin levels fall, causing you to feel less full.

Physical activity declines as we age due to a variety of issues such as tight joints, low energy, and a lack of time. According to research, older persons spend a large portion of their waking hours inactive, ranging from 60 to 80 percent. Lack of activity can have an influence on weight loss attempts.

Maintaining a healthy metabolism is essential for weight management, especially as we age. While conventional wisdom suggests that metabolism slows with age, recent research challenges this assumption. According to research published in the journal Science in 2021, metabolism remains reasonably steady from the ages of 20 to 60 as long as muscle mass does not alter significantly. However, after the age of 60, metabolism slows by around 0.7 percent every year.

Although this drop may appear modest, it can add up over time and have an effect on weight control. Muscle mass is one of the facets that impact metabolism. As we age, we naturally lose muscle mass, which might result in a drop in resting metabolic rate. Resting metabolic rate refers to the number of calories our bodies burn when we are at rest.

Alcohol use might have an effect on weight control and jeopardize your good intentions. Here's how it might alter your appetite and lead to overeating:

· **Increased hunger signals:**

According to research, alcohol can induce hunger signals in the brain, resulting in an increased desire to eat more. This may result in overeating and ingesting more calories than you anticipated.

· **Lower inhibitions:**

Alcohol can lower inhibitions and impair judgment, which may make it more challenging to resist unhealthy food choices or practice portion control. This might lead to eating calorie-dense meals or eating more than you normally would.

· **Empty calories:**

 Alcoholic beverages are frequently heavy in calories yet have little to no nutritional benefit. These calories can add up quickly, especially if you regularly consume alcoholic drinks. It's important to be mindful of the calorie content of your drink choices and consider the impact on your overall calorie intake.

· **Impaired metabolism:**

Alcohol can impair your body's metabolism as well. When alcohol is consumed, the metabolic process prioritizes it, which means that other macronutrients, such as carbs and lipids, may be stored rather than burnt for energy. This may contribute to weight gain in the long run.

4.1: An expert's observation on weight gain

Losing weight becomes more challenging as we age, due to various lifestyle and physiological factors. These factors make it harder to shed a few pounds compared to when we were in our younger or middle age. Some of the factors responsible for this difficulty includes

Arthritis and other conditions:

Certain health conditions like arthritis can impact our stamina, mobility, and balance. These conditions may limit our ability to engage in physical activities and exercise, making weight loss more challenging.

Sleep and stress issues:

As we age, sleep patterns can be disrupted, and stress levels may increase. Lack of quality sleep and chronic stress can affect our metabolism and hormonal balance, making it harder to lose weight.

Dwindling muscle mass:

As we get older, there is a natural decline in muscle mass, known as sarcopenia. Muscle tissue is metabolically active and helps burn calories even at rest. With less muscle mass, our metabolic rate decreases, making weight loss more difficult.

Declining sex hormones:

The levels of sex hormones, such as estrogen and testosterone, decline as we age. These hormones play a role in regulating metabolism and body composition. Their decline can affect our ability to lose weight effectively.

In addition to the previously listed factors, hormones that control fullness and appetite also contribute to the difficulty of maintaining a balanced diet during middle age. Ghrelin and leptin are two important hormones that play a role in this process:

Ghrelin:

Ghrelin is a hormone released by the stomach that stimulates appetite. It signals to the brain that it's time to eat, promoting hunger. Ghrelin levels may alter as we get older, which might lead to more frequent hunger pangs and food cravings. As a result, it could be harder to follow a balanced eating plan and regulate portion amounts.

Leptin:

By reducing hunger, the hormone leptin, which is generated by fat cells, aids in controlling the energy balance. It communicates with the brain to signal fullness and reduce hunger. However, in middle age, leptin sensitivity can decrease, which means the body may not respond as effectively to fullness signals. This can lead to overeating and difficulty in maintaining a healthy eating plan.

4.2: Another expert's view - Reasons why it's Harder to Lose Weight with Age?

The scale is stuck at a place you've never been able to go to or stay below. Although it's annoying, you're not by yourself! Science provides some answers for why our bodies react differently to weight loss efforts as we age. A review by the Agency for Healthcare Research and Quality found that as we age, we naturally tend to gain 1 to 2 pounds (lb) of weight annually. While that might not seem like much, over time it can result in noticeable weight gain and, in certain situations, obesity—defined as having a body mass index (BMI) of 30 or higher—over time.

According to Craig Primack, MD, a specialist in obesity medicine at the Scottsdale Weight Loss Center in Arizona, the prevalence of obesity tends to rise during an individual's twenties, reaching its highest point between the ages of 40 and 59, and thereafter experiencing a little decline after the age of 60. According to Dr. Primack, the likelihood of individuals becoming overweight as they age varies due to factors such as genetic predisposition, degree of physical activity, and dietary preferences. According to the speaker, it is occasionally stated that heredity plays a role in predisposing individuals to certain conditions, while lifestyle choices ultimately determine whether or not these conditions are expressed. Nevertheless, individuals will encounter increasing difficulty in maintaining or reducing body weight as time progresses.

The physiological processes of our muscles, hormones, metabolism, and other bodily systems undergo changes over time as we age. (To put it otherwise, the matter is intricate.) However, it is worth noting that there exist five primary causes that could potentially be attributed to the sensation of increased tightness in one's pants. One is currently undergoing age-related muscle loss. According to an analysis published by the National Institutes of Health (NIH), there is a progressive decrease in lean muscle mass of around 3 to 8 percent per decade after reaching the age of 30. This physiological phenomenon is commonly referred to as sarcopenia. According to Primack, a decrease in physical activity due to age-related health issues like arthritis, or a period of inactivity resulting from accident or surgery, can lead to muscle loss. According to the speaker, while each of these causes may not individually result in a substantial drop, their cumulative impact is indeed significant.

What is the significance of muscle loss in this context? According to the Mayo Clinic, lean muscle has a higher metabolic rate compared to fat, resulting in increased calorie expenditure even during periods of rest. If an individual does not engage in regular weight-based strength training to preserve and enhance muscle mass, their daily caloric requirements will decrease. Continuing to consume the same number of calories as one did in their younger years increases the likelihood of weight gain. According to Marcio Griebeler, MD, an endocrinologist at Cleveland Clinic in

Ohio, the majority of individuals do not often make adjustments to their caloric intake. Individuals consistently consume the same quantity of food; yet, due to a decrease in muscle mass, resulting in a reduced capacity to expend calories, coupled with decreased physical activity levels, they ultimately experience weight increase as time progresses.

The individual is experiencing typical hormonal fluctuations. Based on data obtained from the National Center for Health Statistics, it can be observed that individuals of both genders have alterations in their hormone levels, which contribute to the understanding of why middle age is considered a critical period for weight gain. According to the National Institute on Aging, menopause typically occurs between the ages of 45 and 55 for women. During this period, there is a notable decrease in estrogen levels, leading to the accumulation of excess weight in the abdominal region, as explained by Dr. Griebeler. The alteration in the distribution of adipose tissue can potentially amplify the visibility of weight gain and elevate the susceptibility to hypertension, cardiovascular ailments, hyperlipidemia, and type 2 diabetes.

According to Griebeler, mood swings brought on by hormone fluctuations during perimenopause (the years leading up to menopause) might make it difficult to maintain a good diet and exercise routine. According to UC San Diego Health, as a result, most women put on roughly five pounds as they approach menopause. In contrast, testosterone levels in men naturally decline with age. According to Harvard Health, beyond age 40, it starts to drop at a rate of roughly 1% to 2% year. Testosterone is essential for controlling body fat percentage and maintaining lean muscle mass and strength. If testosterone levels are low, your metabolism may slow down.

According to Harvard Health, growth hormone (GH) production by the pituitary gland decreases with age. Muscle growth and maintenance are among the various roles that GH plays in the body. So, with less GH, it's tougher for your body to develop and retain muscle, which, in turn, also effects how many calories you burn. "It's a snowball effect," Griebeler explains. It's a snowball effect: "You start accumulating more fat, have less lean body mass; you burn fewer calories, and that just keeps adding up over time."

 The Mayo Clinic suggests that losing muscle mass will lower your metabolism, the complex process that transforms the calories in meals into energy. When you have more fat and less muscle, your metabolism slows down. Because of age-related inactivity and other factors, calorie expenditure tends to decline. Age isn't the only factor that impacts your metabolic rate, however - your physical size and sex play a role. Some diseases and disorders, such as hypothyroidism and Cushing's syndrome, tend to be increasingly common as people get older.

Being at the prime of your professional life in your 40s and 50s is fantastic, but it might make it harder to maintain a healthy weight. You might be less active, for one thing. You may spend an hour or more getting to and from work each day, sit at a desk for eight hours or more, and be so busy that you don't have time to go for a walk or exercise. Rachel Lustgarten, RD, a dietitian at Weill Cornell Medicine and New York-Presbyterian Hospital in New York City, points out that if you're too busy to take a lunch break, you're more likely to munch on something from the vending machine or order calorie-dense takeout. Stress from work can also be counterproductive to maintaining a healthy weight. According to a comprehensive review and meta-analysis published in March 2021 in Nutrients, the stress hormone cortisol raises levels of the hormone ghrelin, which makes you eat more.

Some of the factors that contribute to weight increase in middle age have little to do with physiological changes but everything to do with the lifestyle shifts that occur in people's thirties and forties. Having a family is a life-altering experience. Suddenly, you're spending your post-work hour with your child instead of at the gym. Playdates, homework, and other activities will soon fill your child's after-school time. Primack comments, "You don't seem to have time for yourself anymore." As a result, your good intentions to maintain your current weight through food and exercise may suffer.

4.3: How to view Fat?

Body fat is essential for optimal health. However, the environment in which it is stored could potentially impact the likelihood of developing health complications.

Americans are severely overweight. Approximately 42% of men aged 60 and older are obese and have accumulated excess body fat, per the CDC. "However, body fat is not the issue in and of itself, as your body requires a certain amount of fat to remain healthy," explains Dr. Caroline Apovian, co-director of the Center for Weight Management and Wellness at Brigham and Women's Hospital, which is affiliated with Harvard. "Rather, excess stored fat and especially its location in the body have the greatest impact on health."

This is how fat is stored in the body - dietary fat, protein, and carbohydrates are the primary components of food that are primarily metabolized as energy to fuel the fundamental biological processes that sustain life.

Unconsumed fuel is accumulated as lipids (fatty molecules) in adipocytes, which are fat cells distributed throughout the body. In calories, the quantity of this conserved fuel determines the rate of fat cell growth. Fat cells have the capacity to increase or decrease in magnitude by a factor of fifty.

Fat cells remain relatively stable once an individual reaches maturity; they do not undergo any turnover. Additionally, you have no influence over where your body stores fat. "Factors like body type, age, hormones, and genetic predisposition all determine where excess fat ends up," according to Dr. Apovian.

Simply put, stored fat is not harmful. For emergency energy, the body requires fat reserves; fat also insulates and protects vital organs. Additionally, adipocytes secrete leptin, a hormone that functions in the brain to suppress appetite and aid in weight regulation.

Where and how much body fat you possess are critical factors in determining your health. Approximately 90% of body fat in the average person is subcutaneous, or located in a layer just beneath the epidermis. Visceral fat comprises the remaining 10% and is located in the interstitial spaces encompassing the liver, intestines, and other organs, beneath the abdominal wall. Visceral fat is the more problematic of the two: excessive amounts increase the risk of developing type 2 diabetes, cardiovascular disease, and an obese liver. Although fat is present virtually everywhere in the body (chest, back, stomach, glutes), most males - even females also - notice and feel excess fat in the midsection.

Why does adiposity develop? It is not true that consuming fat leads to weight gain; in reality, the opposite may be true. "Many natural foods high in healthy mono- and polyunsaturated fats can make you feel fuller faster because fats are slow to digest," according to Dr. Apovian. She notes that the Mediterranean diet, which was recently ranked as the healthiest diet, is forty percent to fifty percent fat.

Too much caloric intake, regardless of the source, leads to weight gain. Particularly high in calories are ultra-processed foods, including salty munchies, soda, frozen pizza, and fast food. The American Journal of Clinical Nutrition published an online study on October 14, 2021, which found that Americans consume more of them than ever before. The study investigated the daily eating habits of approximately 41,000 adults over a period of 18 years.

Other studies have found that individuals whose diets are high in ultra-processed foods consume approximately 500 additional calories per day in comparison to those whose diets are low in these foods. "The research suggests that ultra-processed foods 'fool' your brain into eating more calories than if you are eating whole foods or unprocessed foods," according to Dr. Apovian. "If your body doesn't use those extra calories, they get stored as fat, and that is why people gain weight."

5.0: 50 and Overweight - the Double Whammy for women

Is the age tag '50' a dampener on your confidence? When you are 50 and overweight, are you the most vulnerable individual in the crowd? What does science say about the presumed susceptibility? Which is more of a problem - the age or the weight?

The phenomenon of women experiencing weight increase during midlife

It is commonly observed that individuals of both genders tend to have a peak in their weight around the age range of 40 to 65, primarily due to a decline in metabolic rate and a decrease in muscle mass. Nevertheless, it is worth noting that women may have a more pronounced increase in body weight compared to men as a result of hormonal fluctuations linked to the onset of menopause.

Despite maintaining their regular habits, numerous women in their forties and fifties frequently experience weight gain and encounter increased difficulty in weight loss endeavors. Based on the findings of Daniela Hurtado, an obesity medicine physician and assistant professor of medicine at Mayo Clinic in Florida, it has been indicated by study that women tend to have an annual weight gain ranging from 0.8 to 1.5 pounds during the midlife phase.

In isolation, Kathleen Jordan, the Chief Marketing Officer (CMO) of Midi Health, a virtual care clinic catering to women aged 40 and beyond, asserted that the hormonal fluctuations experienced during the menopausal transition, characterized by the onset of irregular menstrual cycles, have been linked to an average increase in body weight of approximately six pounds.

A significant factor contributing to the weight increase seen by women after midlife is the decrease in estrogen levels that accompanies menopause. The aforementioned drop has the potential to alter the distribution of adipose tissue in women, impair insulin sensitivity, and elevate levels of cholesterol.

Several studies have also indicated that estrogen may have a potential impact on weight management. In a research study conducted on a cohort of women aged 40 and above, it was shown that those who underwent a pharmacological intervention aimed at inhibiting estrogen production for a duration of 24 weeks experienced a significant increase in adipose tissue, with a mean weight gain exceeding three pounds. A separate investigation revealed that women who were administered estrogen exhibited a higher frequency and intensity of physical exercise compared to those who were prescribed medication that inhibits the effects of estrogen.

According to Wendy Kohrt, a professor of medicine at the University of Colorado Anschutz Medical Campus and the principal researcher on both studies, this observation implies the potential existence of a biological factor contributing to women's weight gain around midlife, rather than solely being influenced by personal choices.

In a study published in the journal EBioMedicine in November, a cohort of more than 600 women was assessed following the consumption of a meal rich in both fat and carbohydrates. Subsequently, the participants were monitored for an additional duration of two weeks. The study revealed that women in the perimenopausal and postmenopausal stages exhibited poorer metabolic health compared to their premenopausal counterparts.

In contrast to premenopausal women, peri- and postmenopausal women had elevated levels of cholesterol and blood pressure, increased glucose and insulin resistance, as well as heightened inflammation. Based on the findings of the study, as reported by Sarah Berry, an associate professor in the department of nutritional sciences at King's College London and the senior author of the study, it was observed that women, regardless of their age, experienced more favorable health outcomes during the premenopausal stage in comparison to the peri- or postmenopausal stages.

5.1: An expert's observation on the issue:

Ineffectiveness in Weight Loss for Women Over the Age of 50 Might Be Due to Hormonal Problems:

In the context of weight loss challenges, hormone-related concerns should almost certainly be regarded as a plausible etiology for weight gain and maintenance in women aged 50 and above.

Certain women have hormonal imbalances that necessitate additional measures beyond adopting a healthier lifestyle to attain weight loss. Hormone issues complicate the already difficult task of weight loss for women over the age of 50; diet and exercise alone will not suffice.

While progesterone and estrogen levels dominate the attention of most women, insufficient testosterone is becoming an increasingly common diagnosis. While low testosterone is more commonly observed in males, it is also possible for women to experience this condition; for women's bodies to operate optimally, all three of these hormones must be in equilibrium.

In the absence of treatment for clinically diagnosed insufficient testosterone, losing weight can be an even more difficult endeavor.

Blood sugar levels can have a substantial effect on the way in which the body functions and feels. Stable blood glucose levels may therefore play a significant role in promoting general health.

Vulnerable bones and joints: reaching postmenopause time to time triggers calcium deficiency leading to feebler frames. In our early years, the body has the ability to substitute the shattered cells with newfangled and robust ones. Nevertheless, with age, this propensity declines where a person has more broken-down cells than substituted ones. Similarly, the joints also turn out to be feeble due to the fact that the tissues and cartilage adjacent to them activate the thinning process gradually.

5.2: Another specialist's take on the women's aging:

1. You might develop a tummy

Reaching your 50s can be a harsh awakening if you've always had an hourglass figure. Even if you continue to work out and eat the same meals as before, your waistline can start to diminish. In order to get ready for pregnancy, estrogen tells your body to store fat in your thighs, buttocks, and breasts. According to Rexrode, "women may notice a shift in their fat distribution - more in the belly rather than on the hips" when estrogen levels drop after menopause. Research indicates that women who are between the ages of 50 and 60 acquire, on average, 1.5 pounds annually.

2. You will be struck harder by alcohol

It is not in your head. The after-dinner cocktail or glass of wine has a greater effect on you as you become older. According to Rexrode, "people get more sensitive to the side effects of alcohol." As you age, your body metabolizes alcohol more slowly. Furthermore, as we age, our muscle mass decreases, leaving less muscle tissue available to assimilate alcohol. In the meanwhile, alcohol may interfere with your drugs, enhancing their effects.

3. You may not be aware of the increased risk of heart disease

Martha Gulati, M.D., a specialist in women's heart disease at Cedars-Sinai Medical Center's Smidt Heart Institute in Los Angeles, says that although heart disease is the leading cause of death for American women, many of them still do not think it is something they should be concerned about. Just 44% of the 1,553 women surveyed in 2019 for the journal Circulation correctly identified heart disease as the top cause of mortality for women in the US.

"They cite breast cancer as their top health concern when we ask them," according to Gulati. "In actuality, women are ten times more likely to die from heart disease than from breast cancer." After menopause, a woman's risk of heart disease increases significantly, and this is also the time that many women first experience the onset of cardiovascular risk factors like high blood pressure or high cholesterol. According to Gulati, following menopause, even women who have always been assured they had low blood pressure may find that it suddenly increases, increasing their risk of suffering a heart attack or stroke.

4. Sexual relations could become awkward

 Low hormone levels after menopause cause the vaginal walls to thin and dry, which can cause discomfort, painful sex, and a decrease in desire, according to urogynecologist Karyn Eilber, M.D. of Cedars-Sinai Medical Center in Los Angeles. Studies reported by the North American Menopause Society indicate that between 17 and 45 percent of postmenopausal women report that they find sex to be uncomfortable. Eilber believes that while the illness is treatable, it's crucial to discuss issues with your spouse and your healthcare practitioner, even though it can be uncomfortable.

5. Your sleeping habits alter

If you've experienced menopause, you may be familiar with how a hot flash may startle you out of a deep sleep and leave you drenched in perspiration. But even after hot flashes pass, ongoing hormonal changes and the rise in body temperature that comes with getting older can affect the length and quality of your sleep, according to Kristin Daley, a psychologist and expert in sleep medicine who serves as the chair of the Society of Behavioral Sleep Medicine's clinical practice committee.

It's possible that you'll wake up more frequently at night or that your sleep will be less peaceful. Furthermore, according to Daley, you won't be able to recover as rapidly following a restless night or if you suffer a time shift when traveling. According to Daley, "our circadian rhythm and our time in bed become more vulnerable to negative influences." You might no longer be that person if you were the one who could fall asleep with the blinds open. We develop extreme sensitivity to light exposure.

6. You develop more fragile bones

Everyone begins to lose some bone density around the age of 50. Menopause, however, causes that bone loss to happen much faster in women. According to some estimates, menopause causes women to lose up to 20% of their bone mass. According to experts, "the drop in estrogen has a very direct effect on bone." This increases the risk of osteoporosis, a disease that weakens bones and can cause fractures, in women. Just one in twenty males over 50 have osteoporosis, compared to approximately one in five women.

Though it's never simple to lose weight, things get much more difficult beyond 50. "In women going through menopause, our estrogen levels drop and our metabolism slows down. Muscle mass is a prerequisite for burning calories, and estrogen increases it. This is according to

Reshmi Srinath, MD, who oversees the Weight and Metabolism Management Program at the Icahn School of Medicine at Mount Sinai in New York. "The main reason it's tougher to lose weight as we age is because hormonal changes are happening for both sexes; men also see a reduction in testosterone after their fourth decade." However, it's not unfeasible.

6.0: Does the Buck stop anywhere?

So, we need to come up with the tackling mechanism for this silent endemic condition. We will explore all the possibilities suggested so far by the seasoned campaigners for weight loss battle.

Before adopting an effective strategy, it will be - nonetheless - wiser to have a look at the different types of diet options we can follow for weight loss journey for any woman over 50.

Catalog of diets

The diet of an individual comprises all food and beverages that are consistently consumed. Dieting refers to the deliberate effort to attain or sustain a specific body weight via dietary means. A variety of factors frequently influence the dietary decisions of individuals, such as clinical necessity, ethical and religious convictions, or a desire to maintain a healthy weight.

Diets that are not considered healthful exist. Certain individuals adhere to unhealthful diets not out of volition but rather as a result of habit. These types of eating patterns are referred to as the "Western diet" and the "junk food diet." Clinicians consider a considerable number of diets to present substantial health hazards with negligible long-term advantages. This is especially true of "fad" or "crash" diets, which are brief weight-loss plans characterized by significant alterations to an individual's typical dietary patterns.

6.1: Diets based on religious beliefs

Religious, spiritual, or philosophical views influence some people's eating choices.

• **Buddhist diet:** While there are no dietary regulations in Buddhism, some Buddhists follow vegetarianism based on

Mahayana Buddhism's rigorous interpretation of the first of the Five Precepts.

• **Hindu diet:** Lacto vegetarian diets are popular among Hindus (though most do not), and are founded on the philosophy of ahimsa (non-harming). Due to cow reverence, eating beef/cattle is forbidden or at the very least taboo among adherents. Most Hindus in India consciously limit their meat consumption in some way.

• **Jain food:** Because of how the Jain faith interprets ahisma, vegetarianism is required for followers; a lacto-vegetarian or vegan diet, in particular, is ideal for Jains. Most Jains also avoid eating root vegetables to avoid injuring insects, worms, and germs when they are removed. Most people also fast in some way. Some Jainists also discourage or prohibit the eating of honey, fungus, alcoholic beverages, and fermented foods.

• **Islamic diet:** Muslims adhere to a diet that consists entirely of halal - allowed in Islam - foods. The inverse of halal is haraam, or Islamically forbidden food. Alcohol, carnivores, pork and other non-ruminant animals, and any flesh from an animal that was not slain using the Islamic manner of ritual slaughter (Dhabiha) are all prohibited. If an otherwise Halal animal was tortured by humans, its meat may nonetheless be considered unfit for Muslims.

• **I-tal:** A system of principles that determines the nutrition of many Rastafari adherents. Natural foods should be ingested, according to one principle. The emphasis is on eating fresh, organic produce that is grown at home or locally. Another concept is to avoid "unclean" foods; this notion is influenced by Biblical teachings. Rastafarians promote teetotalism to conserve "life energy," and many Rastafarians understand I-tal to advocate vegetarianism or veganism as well. Many adherents consider seafood to be a suitable component to an I-tal diet, although they limit the types allowed; fish over a foot long are normally avoided, and all shellfish are avoided because they are not Kosher animals—unlike finned-fish with scales.

• **Kosher diet:** Kosher food is food that is allowed under Kashrut, the set of Jewish dietary restrictions. Some foods and food combinations are not Kosher, and failing to prepare food according to Kashrut can render otherwise legal foods non-Kosher.

• **Seventh-day Adventist diet:** Combines Judaism's Kosher eating regulations with prohibitions on alcoholic beverages and (sometimes) caffeinated beverages. There is a focus on eating whole foods. Meat intake is strongly discouraged but not prohibited; around half of Adventists are lacto-ovo-vegetarians. Vegan and pescetarian diets are also more prevalent among Adventists than among the general public, however many Adventists still eat Kosher meats.

• **Word of Wisdom diet:** The name of a part of the Doctrine and Covenants, a book of scripture recognized by Latter-day Saints. (1) nutritious plants "in the season thereof," (2) eating meat sparingly and only "in times of winter, or of cold, or famine," and (3) grain as the "staff of life." Unlike prohibitions on tobacco, alcohol, coffee, and tea, compliance with meat-avoidance has always been optional among the Church of Jesus Christ of Latter-day Saints, and emphasis on meat-avoidance has largely been withdrawn. According to an official church document, "modern refrigeration methods now make it possible to preserve meat in any season."

6.2: Caloric and weight management diets

The urge to alter food habits is often driven by a desire to reduce weight or to sustain one's current weight. Several weight loss regimens are perceived to include different levels of health hazards, and others are not typically regarded as efficacious. This is particularly accurate when it comes to "crash" or "fad" diets.

Several of the diets mentioned below may fit into multiple subcategories. If this situation occurs, it is explicitly mentioned in the corresponding entry for that specific diet.

6.2.1: Low-calorie diets

The 5:2 diet is a type of intermittent fasting diet.

Intermittent fasting is a dietary approach that involves alternating between periods of not eating and periods of fasting in order to decrease calorie intake.

• **Body for Life:** A diet that focuses on calorie control, which is advocated as part of the 12-week Body for Life program.

• **The cookie diet** is a method of calorie restriction in which individuals consume low-fat cookies to suppress hunger, frequently as a substitute for a meal.

The Hacker's Diet is a calorie-control diet outlined in the book "The Hacker's Diet" by John Walker. The book proposes that the crucial factor in achieving and sustaining the target weight is comprehending and meticulously tracking the intake and expenditure of calories.

• **Nutrisystem diet:** The nutritional component of the weight loss program offered by Nutrisystem, Inc. Nutrisystem delivers meals that are low in calories and have precise proportions of fats, proteins, and carbohydrates.

The Weight Watchers program involves assigning point values to foods, allowing dieters to consume any food as long as they adhere to their daily point restriction.

Consuming fewer than 800 calories on a daily basis is considered to be an extremely low-calorie diet. It is common practice to adhere to such diets while under the guidance of a medical professional. Diets that include no calories are also represented.

• **Inedia,** also known as the breatharian diet, is a diet in which an individual does not consume any food. This diet is based on the concept that prana, rather than food, is required for human survival.

• **The KE diet,** also known as the feeding tube diet, is a type of diet in which an individual does not consume any food while they are fed through a feeding tube.

The Last Chance Diet consists of one low-calorie beverage that is high in protein which will be consumed by the dieter on a daily basis, according to the general assumption. This amounted to a maximum of four hundred calories inside a single day.

On the tongue patch diet, a Marlex patch is stitched to the tongue in order to make eating a painful experience. Therefore, the maximum number of calories that can be consumed in liquid form in a single day is 800.

6.3: carbohydrate-restricted diets

In the latter half of the 20th century and the early 21st century, nutritionist Robert Atkins is credited with popularizing the Atkins diet, which is a low-carbohydrate diet. The proponents of this technique contend that it is a more effective method of weight loss than low-calorie diets, while the detractors contend that a low-carb approach carries higher hazards to one's health. There are four stages that make up the Atkins diet: the Induction phase, the Balancing phase, the Fine-Tuning phase, and the Maintenance phase.

As the patient progresses through the phases, their consumption of carbs gradually increases.

• **The Dukan Diet** is a multi-step diet that emphasizes consuming moderate amounts of carbohydrates and a significant amount of protein. The program begins with two steps that are designed to facilitate weight loss in the short term, and then it moves on to two phases that are designed to consolidate these losses and return to a diet that is more balanced over the long run.

It was discovered that the diet known as **"Kimkins,"** which was aggressively pushed for weight loss, was a scam.

• **The South Beach Diet** is a diet that was designed by a cardiologist named Arthur Agatston, who is located in Miami. According to Agatston, the key to losing weight quickly and being healthy is not eliminating all carbohydrates and fats from one's diet, but rather selecting the appropriate carbohydrates and fats to consume.

• **The Stillman diet** is a carbohydrate-restricted diet that was developed prior to the Atkins diet and allows for the eating of particular food components.

6.4: Low-fat diets

• McDougall's starch diet is a high-fiber, low-fat, high-calorie diet based on starches such as potatoes, rice, and legumes; it excludes added vegetable oils and animal products. John A. McDougall's analysis is informed by historical observations that demonstrate the prevalence of starch-based diets among civilizations across the globe.

6.5: Intensive diets

Crash diets are diets that are extremely low in calories and are used with the objective of losing weight very quickly. They are used to disparage popular eating behaviors that are regarded to be unhealthy, but they are also used to characterize diet regimens that include making significant and rapid alterations to the amount of food that is consumed. Without the supervision of a medical professional, this diet is extremely risky and has the potential to result in an unexpected death.

- **The Beverly Hills Diet** is a rigorous eating plan that begins with a consumption of only fruits for the first few days and then gradually expands the range of foods consumed until the sixth week.

• **The cabbage soup diet** is a low-calorie diet that emphasizes increasing the amount of cabbage soup that one consumes. Considered to be a trendy diet.

• **The grapefruit diet** is a popular diet that is associated with the goal of facilitating weight loss. This diet involves the consumption of significant quantities of grapefruit during meal times.

• **A monotrophic diet** is a diet that consists of consuming only one food item or one type of food for a specific amount of time in order to achieve the targeted weight loss.

One type of crash diet is known as **the Subway diet,** which involves consuming sandwiches from Subway rather than other fast foods that are higher in calories. The convicted sexual offender and previously obese student Jared Fogle, who shed 245 pounds by substituting his meals with Subway sandwiches as part of his endeavor to lose weight, is credited with making this product famous.

6.6: Reset eating plans

On **detox diets**, you either cut out or try to eliminate substances that you think are bad for you. Some examples include limiting your food intake to items that do not contain any artificial colors or preservatives, increasing your water consumption, or taking nutritional supplements. Because hyponatremia can occur from consuming far more water than what is suggested, the second technique in particular has come under fire. We call detox diets "pseudoscience" because we can't find any proof that they work.

• **Juice fasting:** a cleansing regimen in which one drinks only juices of fruits and vegetables for sustenance. There is debate on the effects of these diets on health.

• **Master Cleanse:** a juice fast with a twist that calls for tea and lemonade instead of food.

6.7: Diets that are followed from a medical standpoint

When people have intolerances or allergies to particular kinds of food, it can sometimes influence the decisions they make regarding their diet. In addition, there are dietary patterns that may be recommended, prescribed, or supplied by medical practitioners to those who have particular medical requirements.

• **The Dietary Approaches to Stop Hypertension (DASH)** diet is a recommendation that those who have high blood pressure consume a diet that is mostly composed of fruits, vegetables, whole grains, and dairy products with a low-fat content. Additionally, it is recommended that individuals with high blood pressure avoid meals that are sweetened with sugar, red meat, and fats. Promoted by the United States Department of Health and Human Services, which is an organization that is part of the United States government.

The term **"diabetic diet"** refers to a broad category of diets that are recommended to individuals who have diabetes. Within the scientific world, there is a significant amount of dispute over the type of diet that is most beneficial for individuals who have diabetes.

• **The elemental diet** is a medical diet that consists solely of liquids and emphasizes the consumption of fluids in order to facilitate easier digestion.

Through the process of elimination, an elimination diet is a procedure that can be used to determine which foods are responsible for unfavorable effects in a person.

A diet that does not contain gluten, which is a protein that can be found in barley, rye, and wheat, is referred to as a gluten-free diet. Gluten-related illnesses, such as coeliac disease, non-celiac gluten sensitivity, gluten ataxia, dermatitis herpetiformis, and wheat allergy, are one of the conditions that can be treated with this medicinal intervention.

Gluten-free and casein-free diet: a diet that does not contain gluten and also does not contain casein, which is a protein that is typically present in dairy products and cheese. Research has been conducted to determine whether or not this diet is effective in treating autism spectrum disorder.

Those who are afflicted with chronic kidney disease, those who have only one kidney, those who have a kidney infection, and those who may be suffering from some other form of kidney failure are the individuals who should adhere to the healthy kidney diet. The food that is used for dialysis is not the same as this diet; it is entirely different. Not only does the healthy renal diet prohibit significant amounts of protein, which is difficult for the kidney to break down, but it also restricts foods and beverages that are rich in potassium and phosphorus. Consumption of liquids is frequently restricted as well.

• **The ketogenic diet is** a high-fat, low-carb diet that encourages the conversion of both nutritional fat and body fat into usable energy. It is a medical medication that is utilized for the treatment of refractory epilepsy.

The term "liquid diet" refers to a diet in which you consume nothing but liquids. The administration of this medication by physicians may be necessary for medical reasons, such as following a gastric bypass or to prevent death from starvation as a result of a hunger strike.

The low-FODMAP diet is a type of diet that prevents the consumption of all fermentable carbohydrates (FODMAPs) on a worldwide scale.

• **Soft diet:** A mechanical soft diet, also known as an edentulous diet, or soft food(s) diet, is a diet that consists solely of foods that are physically soft. The purpose of this diet is to reduce or eliminate the need to chew the meal. People who have difficulty chewing food, such as those who have certain types of dysphagia (difficulty swallowing), the loss of many or all of their teeth, pain from newly adjusted dental braces, or surgery involving the jaw, mouth, or gastrointestinal tract, are suggested to use this product.

One type of diet is known as the specific carbohydrate diet, and its primary objective is to limit the consumption of complex carbs, which can be found in grains and complex sugars.

6.8: Fad diets

A fad diet refers to a diet that gains temporary popularity, akin to fashion trends, but is not considered a conventional nutritional guideline. These diets often make unrealistic claims of rapid weight loss or illogical health benefits. A fad diet lacks a specific definition and includes a range of diets that have diverse methodologies, evidence bases, and consequently, varying outcomes, benefits, and drawbacks. Additionally, fad diets are always evolving. In general, fad diets offer quick but temporary results with no exertion, often failing to educate individuals about the comprehensive dietary and lifestyle modifications required for long-lasting health advantages. Fad diets are sometimes endorsed with hyperbolic assertions, such as the attainment of quick weight loss exceeding 1 kg per week or the enhancement of health through "detoxification," or even dangerous assertions.

Due to the ever-changing nature of the "fad" designation, influenced by social, cultural, and subjective factors, it is impossible to provide a comprehensive list. Fad diets, including the Mediterranean diet, may either persist or cease to be considered fads. Certain conditions, such as epilepsy or obesity, may benefit from certain diets with therapeutic purposes. However, there is no universally effective diet that guarantees weight loss or improved appearance for all individuals. Dieticians are a profession that is subject to regulation and can differentiate between nutritionally balanced diets and those that are detrimental to health.

6.8.1: Diets that are particular to foods

• **The alkaline diet:** The alkaline diet, also known as the alkaline ash diet, the alkaline acid diet, the acid ash diet, and the acid alkaline diet, is a series of diets that are loosely related to one another. These diets are based on the misunderstanding that certain kinds of food can have an influence on the pH balance of the body. The acid ash hypothesis, which was mostly associated with osteoporosis research, was the source of conception for this idea. Supporters of the diet are of the opinion that particular foods have the potential to influence the acidity (pH) of the body, and that this change in pH can consequently be utilized for the purpose of treating or preventing disease. On the other hand, their assertions are not true, and there is no proof to back up the mechanisms that are claimed to be associated with this diet, which is not suggested by dietitians or any other kinds of health specialists.

• Baby food diet: Baby food is any food that is soft and readily swallowed, other than breastmilk or infant formula, and is designed specifically for human infants between the ages of six months and two years (the age range of baby food). It is possible that the meal is table food that is consumed by the family and has been mashed or otherwise broken down. The food is available in a wide variety of tastes and variations, and it can be purchased ready-made from producers.

• **Cabbage soup diet:** The cabbage soup diet is a revolutionary weight loss program that focuses on the intake of a low-calorie cabbage soup in large quantities over the course of seven days. It is typically believed to be a fad diet due to the fact that it is intended for weight loss in the short term and does not demand any commitment with regard to the long term.

- Carnivore diet: Meat, eggs, and dairy products are the only foods that are allowed to be taken on the carnivore diet, which is also known as a zero-carb diet. This diet is a trend that gained popularity in recent years. The carnivore diet is linked to health claims that are not supported by true scientific evidence. It is possible for such a diet to result in deficits of vitamins and dietary fiber, as well as an increase in the frequency of chronic diseases. Only beef is allowed to be consumed on the lion diet, which is a variation of the carnivore diet that is extremely restrictive.

• **Clean eating:** clean eating is a fad diet that is based on the assumption that there are specific health benefits associated with consuming whole foods and avoiding convenience meals and other processed foods. There are various variations of the diet that urge the intake of raw food and may exclude gluten, grains, and/or dairy products. There is a lack of scientific evidence to support extreme variations of the diet, which has led to criticism that these variations may pose possible health hazards.

• **Cookie diet:** A cookie diet is a calorie-restricted fad diet that is supposed to produce weight loss. It is centered on meal replacement in the shape of a cookie that has been carefully created.

The egg and wine diet: this is a fad diet that gained popularity in 1964 and has been revived in 2018 on social media platforms. The diet is a combination of eating eggs and drinking wine.

In 2018, the diet was brought back to life on various social media sites, where it emerged as a meme. The diet has been criticized by professionals in the medical field since it is not only unsustainable but also nutritionally unbalanced, and it will, in the long run, cause more harm than benefit. The diet has been characterized as hazardous and a potential risk to the liver due to the significant amount of alcohol that it contains.

A nutritional approach that involves the deliberate consumption of specific food types either together or separately is referred to as the food combining diet. In the case of weight control regimens, for instance, it is recommended that carbs and proteins not be ingested at the same meal.

When following **the Fit for Life diet,** it is recommended that you do not combine carbohydrates and proteins, that you do not drink water at mealtimes, and that you stay away from dairy products.

• **Fruitarianism:** it is a diet that does not include any items derived from animals and consists mostly on the consumption of fruits, with the possibility of also including nuts and seeds. Fruitarian diets have been the subject of criticism and worries over their health.

• Although **the gluten-free diet** is necessary for individuals who suffer from celiac disease or gluten sensitivity, it has also become a trend in recent years.

• **The Grapefruit Diet:** The Grapefruit Diet, sometimes referred to as the Hollywood Diet and the 18-Day Diet, is a diet that is meant to be followed for a limited amount of time. In general, it entails consuming one grapefruit at each meal, in addition to meat, eggs, and other meals that are high in fat and protein, as well as specific veggies. As a result, the grapefruit diet is a diet that is low in carbohydrates. After a period of ten to twelve days, the grapefruit diet is followed by a break of two days.

• **The Lamb Chop and Pineapple Diet:** The Lamb Chop and Pineapple Diet was a high-protein fad diet that was popular in the United States during the 1920s. It was hypothesized that pineapples would supply an adequate amount of sugar for energy, while lamb chops would supply an adequate amount of protein for strength. Furthermore, the fruit acid would either absorb or eliminate any fat that was left over from the lamb chops.

• **Macrobiotics:** A macrobiotic diet, often known as a macrobiotic diet, is a trend diet that utilizes concepts regarding different kinds of food that are derived from Zen Buddhism. The dietary plan is an attempt to strike a balance between the yin and yang aspects of food and cooking utensils. One of the most important tenets of macrobiotic diets is to limit the use of animal products, to consume foods that are cultivated locally and are in season, and to consume meals in moderation.

• **The Morning Banana Diet:** The Morning Banana Diet is a fad diet that gained popularity in Japan in 2008 and began to gain some traction in the Western world following that year. As part of the diet plan, you are permitted to consume an unrestricted number of bananas with either a portion of milk or water at room temperature for breakfast. According to nutritionists, "a healthy person can consume at least seven and a half bananas before reaching the recommended level" of potassium, which is a dietary mineral that is found in bananas. This is despite the fact that the diet legally permits an unrestricted consumption of bananas. The menu options for lunch and dinner are completely unrestricted. Between meals, users are permitted to consume one or more bananas as a snack; however, they are not permitted to consume any other sweets. There is no food allowed after eight o'clock, and the dieter is required to go to bed by midnight.

Depending on the context, the term **"Paleolithic diet"** can refer to either the eating patterns that people followed throughout the Paleolithic period or to contemporary diet regimens that claim to be based on ancient eating patterns.

A plant-based diet that combines the ideas of the paleo diet and the vegan diet is referred to as the **Pegan Diet**. The Pegan diet does not contain gluten and also promotes the intake of vegetables that do not contain carbohydrate, as well as grass-fed organic meats and fish that is low in mercury. 75% of the diet is comprised of plant-based foods, and the only fruits that are allowed are low-glycemic berries. On the Pegan diet, refined sugar and items that can cause an increase in insulin production are abstained from. The diet is also against cow's milk, although it does not exclude dairy products. The occasional use of organic goat or sheep milk, yogurt, kefir, grass-fed butter, ghee, or cheese is permitted on this occasion.

Superfood is a marketing phrase for food that is said to bestow health benefits as a result of an unusual nutritional density. The superfood diet is just one example of this marketing term. It is not normal practice for nutrition scientists, dietitians, and other specialists to use this word. The majority of these individuals are of the opinion that certain foods do not possess the health benefits that these supporters assert they do. Many new, exotic, and foreign fruits or ancient grains are marketed under the phrase – or superfruit or supergrain respectively – after being introduced or re-introduced to Western markets. This is the case even if there is no scientific evidence to support the claim that these fruits or grains contain exceptional levels of nutrients.

• **Whole30 diet:** The Whole30 diet is a type of elimination diet that is followed for a period of thirty days and places an emphasis on eating whole foods while excluding sugar, alcohol, wheat, and dairy products. Additionally, beans and soy are not allowed to be consumed during the original Whole30 diet, although a plant-based variation of the Whole30 diet permits the eating of these food categories. In the classic Whole30 diet, members are not permitted to consume natural sweeteners such as honey or maple syrup, which results in a diet that is comparable to the paleo diet but more stringent. In addition, there has been a limited amount of independent study done on the Whole30 diet, and there is no scientific proof to support the health claims that Whole30 makes.

6.8.2: High-fat diets with a low carbohydrate intake
• **Low-carbohydrate diet:** In comparison to the typical diet, low-carbohydrate diets limit the amount of carbohydrates that are consumed. Foods that are high in carbohydrates, such as sugar, bread, and pasta, are restricted and replaced with foods that contain a higher percentage of fat and protein, such as meat, poultry, fish, shellfish, eggs, cheese, nuts, and seeds, as well as foods that are low in carbohydrates, such as spinach, kale, chard, collards, and other fibrous vegetables.

• **The Atkins diet:** The Atkins diet is a low-carbohydrate fad diet that was developed by Robert Atkins in the 1970s. It was marketed with claims that restricting carbohydrates is crucial to weight loss and that the diet offered "a high-calorie way to stay thin forever."

• Bulletproof diet: The Bulletproof diet, which was designed and promoted by Asprey, requires individuals to consume foods that are high in fat, moderate in protein, and low in carbohydrates. The consumption of Bulletproof Coffee, which is a brand of coffee that is manufactured and marketed by Asprey, serves as the basis for the Bulletproof diet. After spending time in Tibet and consuming yak-butter tea, Asprey came up with the recipe for his Bulletproof Coffee in the process. After his return to the United States, he began experimenting with other recipes for buttered beverages. In 2009, he posted the recipe for his buttered coffee drink on his blog. Soy, wheat, canned veggies, and meals that have been microwaved are all considered to be harmful according to the Bulletproof diet, which encourages the intake of grass-fed beef and butter. Furthermore, it suggests introducing intermittent fasting into your routine.

The original ketogenic diet, often known as **the "keto" diet,** is a diet that is rich in fat and low in carbohydrates. It was established in the 1920s and was initially used to treat drug-resistant epilepsy in children. The diet that has become popular and has taken on the same name is similarly a diet that is heavy in fat and low in carbohydrates, but it claims to cause weight loss. When the body is deprived of glucose, which is gained from foods that are high in carbohydrates, the ketogenic diet for weight loss is based on the idea that the body would manufacture energy from fat that has been stored. Approximately fifty percent of the food consumed on this ketogenic diet for adults is composed of fat, which accounts for seventy percent of the total calories.

• **Protein Power:** The concept behind Protein Power is that lowering the amount of carbs that are consumed will result in a decrease in the amount of insulin that is introduced into the body. Insulin, which is triggered by the consumption of carbs, is said to be responsible for controlling the storage of fat through the eating process. A diet that is based on animals and is abundant in red meat and eggs is encouraged by Protein Power. There is no evidence from scientific research to support the claims made about the diet.

It has been said that Protein Power is a diet that is a craze and that it is pseudoscientific. Diets that are high in protein, such as Protein Power, may be useful for achieving temporary weight loss through the restriction of calories, but they are not effective for achieving long-term weight control.

• **Sugar Busters:** The Sugar Busters diet is a diet that focuses on avoiding foods that include refined carbohydrates such as refined sugar, white flour, and white rice. Additionally, the Sugar Busters diet eliminates naturally occurring carbs that have a high glycemic index, such as potatoes and carrots.

• **The zone diet** is a type of diet in which a person makes an effort to divide their calorie intake into three categories: carbohydrates, proteins, and fats, with the ratio of 40:30:30.

• **Scarsdale medical diet:** This diet is comparable to the Atkins Diet and the Stillman Diet in that it stresses the need of consuming a diet that is rich in protein and low in carbohydrates. Additionally, it places an emphasis on the consumption of fruits and vegetables. On the other hand, the diet permits an unlimited quantity of animal protein, particularly eggs, fish, lean meats, and poultry. Certain items are banned while others are allowed. The diet suggests that on Sundays, one should consume "plenty of steak" along with vegetables such as tomatoes, celery, or brussels sprouts. Between seven and fourteen days is the duration of the Scarsdale diet, which is a low-calorie diet that limits daily calorie intake to a maximum of one thousand.

• **The South Beach Diet:** This diet is comprised of three stages, and as it proceeds, the amount of carbohydrates ingested steadily increases while at the same time the proportions of fat and protein consumed decrease. Furthermore, it incorporates a concept of "good" fats, which are primarily monounsaturated, and contains a variety of items that are suggested, such as vegetables and lean meats. It does not place any restrictions on the number of calories that are consumed, it incorporates a workout routine, and it is based on the principle of eating three main meals and two snacks each day.

6.8.3: Low-fat diets that are high in carbohydrates

• **Ornish diet:** Ornish has advocated for a meal plan that is commonly referred to as the "Ornish diet" in order to both prevent and reverse heart disease. Because it allows for the use of egg whites and dairy products that are low in fat, the Ornish diet is considered to be lacto-ovo vegetarian. When following the Ornish diet, it is strictly banned to consume any and all meat, fish, poultry, fat dairy products, coconuts, margarine, nuts, seeds, avocados, olives, and cooking oils (with the exception of canola oil). The diet is free of cholesterol and contains only ten percent of total calories that come from fat. It is also very low in fat. A significant emphasis is placed on the consumption of fruits, legumes, vegetables, and whole grains within the Ornish diet.

A low-fat fad diet is what **the McDougall diet** is, according to the classification system. Not only does the diet prohibit all goods derived from animals, but it also prohibits cooking oils, processed foods, alcoholic beverages, and caffeinated beverages. Flatulence, perhaps poor mineral absorption from extra fiber, and limited food options that may contribute to a feeling of deprivation are all potential side effects of this eating plan, just as they are with any other restrictive diet that is high in fiber.

• The **Primakin Diet** is a nutrition plan that emphasizes the intake of foods that have not been processed.

6.8.4: Fluid-based diets

• Diets that are primarily composed of liquids, also known as soft "foods" that dissolve at room temperature (like ice cream), are referred to as **liquid diets**. In general, a liquid diet helps provide adequate hydration, contributes to the maintenance of electrolyte balance, and is frequently prescribed for individuals in situations where solid food diets are not recommended. This includes individuals who suffer from gastrointestinal illness or damage, as well as individuals who undergo certain types of medical tests or surgeries that involve the mouth or the digestive tract.

• **SlimFast:** SlimFast is an American corporation with its headquarters in Palm Beach Gardens, Florida. The company is responsible for marketing an eponymous brand of shakes, bars, snacks, packed meals, and other dietary supplement items. These products are available in the United States of America, Canada, France, Germany, Iceland, Ireland, Latin America, and a number of other countries. A number of diets and weight loss regimes that feature SlimFast's meal products are promoted by the company.

6.9: Observing a fast

• The 5:2 Diet is a sort of periodic fasting that does not adhere to a specific eating pattern and places an emphasis solely on the number of calories consumed. To put it another way, two days of the week are dedicated to the consumption of roughly 500 to 600 calories, which is equivalent to approximately 25 percent of the typical daily caloric intake. The remaining five days of the week are committed to the consumption of normal amounts of calories.

• **Breatharian diet:** A diet that is based on the concept that individuals can survive just on spirituality and sunlight, yet it leads to famine, and believers have been seen eating and drinking while they are hiding.

• **Intermittent fasting:** Intermittent fasting refers to any of the many different meal timing regimens that alternate between periods of non-fasting and periods of deliberate fasting (or limited calorie intake) throughout the course of a certain time period. Alternate-day fasting, periodic fasting like the 5:2 diet, and daily time-restricted eating (TRE) are all examples of some of the methods that fall under the category of intermittent fasting.

• **Juice fasting:** Juice fasting, also known as juice cleaning, is a trend diet in which a person drinks only juices made from fruits and vegetables while avoiding the ingestion of solid foods entirely. Detoxification, which is a treatment used in alternative medicine, is what it is used for, and it is frequently included in detox diets. The diet can normally last anywhere from one to seven days and includes a variety of fruits and vegetables, as well as spices, that are not typically included in the juices that are marketed or consumed in the typical Western diet. In other cases, the diet is advertised with claims that are not only improbable but also unsupported about the health benefits it offers.

• **Orthopathy:** Orthopathy, also known as natural hygiene (NH), is a collection of alternative medical ideas and practices that originated from the Nature Cure movement. All that is required to prevent and treat disease, according to proponents, is to make changes to one's lifestyle, such as fasting, dieting, and other lifestyle choices.

The protein-sparing modified fast, also known as **the PSMF diet**, is a type of diet that is considered to be very low in calories, with a daily calorie intake of less than 800. This diet is characterized by a high proportion of protein calories, while simultaneously restricting carbohydrate and fat intake levels. The addition of vitamins and minerals, as well as the inclusion of a protein component, are all included. PSMF diets can persist for up to six months, after which there is a progressive increase in the number of calories consumed over a period of six to eight weeks.

6.10: Detoxifying the body

The term **"detox diet"** refers to a type of diet plan that asserts to have the ability to bring about detoxification. Contaminants are substances that are considered to be unneeded for human life. These substances include flavor enhancers, food colorings, pesticides, and preservatives. However, the overall idea suggests that the majority of food contains contaminants. Scientists, dietitians, and medical professionals, despite the fact that they typically consider brief "detox diets" to be harmless (unless they result in nutritional deficit), frequently question the utility and necessity of "detox diets" due to a lack of supporting factual evidence or coherent rationale. In situations where a person is suffering from a condition, the notion that a detox diet is effective can cause them to delay or even forego seeking therapy that is effective from the beginning.

• **The lemon detox diet** is a modified version of the juice fast that discourages the consumption of food and instead encourages the consumption of tea and lemonade that is flavored with maple syrup and cayenne pepper. The proponents of the diet assert that it cleanses, reduces, and tones the body, which in turn enables the body to cure itself independently. The diet does not appear to eliminate any toxins, nor does it appear to do anything other than a brief reduction of weight, which is then quickly regained. There is no data to support any of these claims.

6.11: Diets that are vegetarian

If you don't eat any meat, you're following a vegetarian diet. Furthermore, vegetarians abstain from consuming foods that include by-products of animal slaughter, such as gelatin and rennet that are derived from animals.

The term **"fruitarian diet"** refers to a form of eating that focuses mostly on eating fresh fruit.

• **Lacto vegetarianism** is a sort of vegetarian diet that allows for the use of some types of dairy products, but is not permitted to consume eggs or items that contain animal rennet. a diet that adherents of a number of religions, including Jainism, Sikhism, and Hinduism, follow in accordance with the principle of Ahimsa, which means "non-harming without harming."

• **Ovo vegetarianism** is a type of vegetarian diet that does not include dairy products but does contain eggs.

The term "ovo-lacto vegetarianism" refers to a vegetarian diet that incorporates dairy products and eggs.

Vegans, in addition to abstaining from the foods that are included in a vegetarian diet, do not consume any items that are derived from animals. This includes products such as eggs, dairy products, and honey. The vegan ideology and lifestyle encompass more than just the diet; it also involves avoiding the use of any products that have been tested on animals and frequently advocating for the rights and welfare of animals.

6.12: A diet that is semi-vegetarian

The term **"semi-vegetarianism"** refers to a diet that is primarily vegetarian but does allow for the consumption of meat on occasion. Diets such as **"flexitarian,"** **"reducetarian,"** and **"demitarian"** are included in this category. Sometimes, semi-vegetarian and flexitarian diets are regarded as being distinct from one another. For example, the former is defined as excluding red meat, while the latter just involves eating meat on a less frequent basis.

• **Pescetarianism** is a diet that consists of seafood but excludes poultry, other white meat, and meat from mammals but does contain seafood.

The term **"pollotarianism"** refers to a diet that excludes all other types of white meat, seafood, and meat from animals, but does include chicken.

The Kangatarian diet is a type of diet that originated in Australia. Kangaroo meat is ingested in addition to the items that are allowed to be consumed by vegetarians through a vegetarian diet. Rather than being a dietary word or distinguishing label that was ever intended to be taken seriously or utilized in a manner that was not humorous, the name is a protologism that may have originated as a joke.

Planetary health diets are dietary paradigms that have the following goals: to feed a growing population throughout the world, to significantly reduce the number of fatalities that are caused by poor diets around the world, and to be environmentally sustainable in order to prevent the collapse of the natural world.

• A plant-based diet is a broad word that is used to describe diets in which consumption of animal products does not constitute a significant percentage of the diet. It is possible to follow a plant-based diet while occasionally consuming meat, according to certain definitions of the term. Other definitions, on the other hand, consider a plant-based diet to be completely vegetarian.

6.13: The other diets

• An alkaline diet is a diet that involves avoiding foods that are relatively acidic, or foods that have a low pH level. These foods include things like alcohol, caffeine, dairy products, fungus, grains, meat, and sugar. Others who advocate for such a diet feel that it might be beneficial to one's health, while others who oppose it believe that the claims lack any scientific validity.

 Eating in a clean manner:

• **The climatarian diet** is a diet that focuses on decreasing the carbon footprint of the food that is consumed, primarily through the consumption of food that is sourced locally and the avoidance of beef and lamb meat. Also, adherents may be "organivores," which are those who strongly choose certified organic foods over meals that are produced through intensive farming.

• **The Eat-Clean Diet** is a diet that emphasizes the consumption of foods that do not contain any preservatives and the combination of lean proteins and complex carbs.

• **Germ therapy** is a sort of alternative medicine that entails following a diet that is low in salt, low in fat, and vegetarian. Additionally, the diet requires the consumption of particular supplements. Max Gerson, the original developer of the therapy, asserted that it had the potential to treat cancer as well as other chronic and degenerative diseases. This assertion has not been substantiated by scientific evidence, and it has the potential to result in severe sickness and even death.

• **The Graham Diet** is a vegetarian diet that encourages the intake of whole-wheat flour and discourages the consumption of stimulants like alcohol and caffeine. During the 19th century, Sylvester Graham was the one who developed it.

A food-combining diet that was devised by William Howard Hay in the 1920s is referred to as **the Hay diet.** Foods are separated into their respective categories, and it is recommended that carbs and proteins not be ingested at the same meal.

The term **"high-protein diet"** refers to a diet that is designed to increase muscle mass by consuming a significant amount of protein. These diets should not be confused with low-carb diets, which aim to reduce the amount of carbohydrates consumed in order to achieve weight loss.

The term **"high residue diet"** refers to a diet that emphasizes the consumption of a significant amount of dietary fibre. Certain types of fruits, vegetables, nuts, and grains are examples of foods that are high in fiber.

Walrus meat that has been frozen and matured is distributed among **Inuit** families.

Inuit people traditionally eat food that is obtained by fishing, hunting, or gathering in the area, with the majority of their diet consisting of meat and fish.

One of the weight loss programs offered by Jenny Craig, Inc. is called **Jenny Craig**. A number of components are included, one of which is weight counseling. One of the dietary aspects involves the eating of food that has been pre-packaged and manufactured by the corporation.

• **The locavore diet is** a neologism that describes the consumption of food that is produced locally and is not transported for a significant distance to reach the market. An illustration of this can be seen in the book "100-Mile Diet," in which the writers devoted an entire year to consuming only food that was farmed within a radius of one hundred miles from their place of residence. Locavores are a term that is occasionally used to refer to individuals who adhere to this type of diet.

The term **"low carbon diet"** refers to the consumption of food that has been produced, processed, and delivered with a minimum of greenhouse gas emissions linked from the production process.

The term **"low-fat diet"** refers to a diet that restricts fat consumption, and in many cases, it also restricts cholesterol and saturated fat consumption. The purpose of diets that are low in fat is to lessen the likelihood of developing illnesses such as obesity and cardiovascular disease. Since the composition of macronutrients does not play a role in determining whether or not a diet is successful in terms of weight loss, they behave similarly to a diet that is low in carbohydrates. To put that into perspective, carbs and protein each contribute four calories per gram, whereas fat contributes nine calories per gram. For the purpose of regulating the amount of saturated fat consumed, the Institute of Medicine suggests limiting fat consumption to 35 percent of total calories.

• Diets with a low glycemic index, often known as low-carbohydrate diets, are diets that limit the amount of carbohydrates consumed in comparison to the typical diet. Foods that are high in carbohydrates, such as sugar, bread, and pasta, are restricted and replaced with foods that contain a higher percentage of fat and protein, such as meat, poultry, fish, shellfish, eggs, cheese, nuts, and seeds, as well as foods that are low in carbohydrates, such as spinach, kale, chard, collards, and other fibrous vegetables.

The term "low-protein diet" refers to a consumption pattern in which individuals reduce the amount of protein that they consume. It is possible to use a diet low in protein as a treatment for metabolic illnesses that are hereditary, such as phenylketonuria and homocystinuria. Additionally, using a diet low in protein can be utilized to treat kidney or liver disease. Alterations in calcium homeostasis are likely to be responsible for the reduction in bone fracture risk that is observed in individuals who consume a low amount of protein. Therefore, there is no universally accepted definition of what defines low-protein. This is due to the fact that the quantity and composition of protein for an individual with phenylketonuria would be significantly different from that of an individual with homocystinuria or tyrosinemia.

• **A macrobiotic diet** is a healthy eating plan that does not include any processed foods. The following are examples of common components: grains, beans, and vegetables.

The term **"Mediterranean diet"** refers to a diet that is based on the eating habits of regions in southern Europe. Olive oil serves as the principal source of fat, which is one of the characteristics that sets it apart from other ingredients.

The DASH diet and the Mediterranean diet are combined into **the MIND diet**, which is a combination of the two. The diet is designed to slow the progression of neurological symptoms, such as those associated with Alzheimer's disease.

A weight-loss diet that is characterized by the use of carbohydrates that have a low glycemic index is known as **the Montignac diet**.

• **Mushroom diet:** a diet that is primarily composed of mushrooms.

One of the claims made by numerous weight-loss programs is that certain foods, like celery, require more calories to digest than they really offer. This is known as **the negative calorie diet**. This assertion is based on a questionable foundation.

A diet that is low in calories and is based on the typical eating patterns of people who live in the Ryukyu Islands is known as **the Okinawa diet**.

• **Omnivorous diet:** An omnivore is someone who consumes a wide variety of foods that come from both plant and animal sources.

The organic food diet is a diet that consists solely of organic food, which means that the food has not been produced using any modern inputs, such as synthetic fertilizers, genetic modification, irradiation, antibiotics, growth hormones, or synthetic food additives.

Inmates who are not trusted to handle utensils are provided with a meal alternative known as "prison loaf" in certain correctional facilities in the United States. It is meant to give convicts with all of their dietary requirements, although its composition differs from institution to institution and state to state. However, it is intended to serve as a replacement for conventional meals.

• **Raw foodism** is a dieting approach that emphasizes the eating of food that has not been cooked or processed in any way. Raw food diets are frequently linked with vegetarian diets; nevertheless, there are raw meat diets that include raw meat consumption.

• **The Shangri-La Diet:** The Shangri-La Diet is both the name of a book written by the psychologist Seth Roberts, who is a professor at Tsinghua University and a professor emeritus at UC Berkeley, as well as the name of the diet that is advocated in the book. A method of hunger suppression that can lead to weight loss is discussed in the book. This method involves taking 100–400 calories per day in a flavorless food, such as extra light olive oil, one hour outside of mealtimes.

• **Slimming World diet:** Slimming World is a weight loss organization that helps men and women of all ages lose weight. The organization's headquarters are located in Derbyshire, England. The primary objective of the program is weight loss, and once members have achieved their desired weight, they are provided with support to help them maintain a healthy weight. A network of 3,500 "consultants" located all throughout the country is used to carry out its operations. In addition to providing a group support service known as IMAGE Therapy, Slimming World provides an eating plan that is based on the satiety and energy density of the food that is consumed.

A diet that emphasizes the consumption of **"power foods"** and is based on controlling portion sizes is known as the Sonoma diet.

• Diet of the SparkPeople

The consumption of refined carbohydrates, and sugars in particular, is the primary focus of this lifestyle modification.

In many industrialized countries, particularly those in the Anglosphere, the "default" diet is **the Western pattern diet**, sometimes known as the WPD. It is commonly referred to as the **"meat-sweet diet"** due to the high consumption of meat (overall), red meats (especially), dairy products, sweets, and refined cereals. The phrase originates from the "Western world" and is interchangeable with the "standard American diet." For the most part, people consume an inadequate number of whole grains, legumes, tree nuts, fruit, and fish. The weight loss diet (WPD) is distinguished from other unbalanced diets by the heavy inclusion of "junk food" and other ultra-processed foods that typically provide substantial amounts of empty calories, net carbs, simple carbs, saturated fat, industrial trans-fat, added sugar/free sugars, added salt, artificial flavor/sweetener, and other processing ingredients. Typical examples include ready-to-eat cereals, white breads, fast food, other convenience meals, cured meat dishes, smoked or fried meats, fried dough foods, shallow or deep-fried potatoes, other foods that are intensely fried in rendered fat or refined oil, sugary or fatty discretionary foods (such as sauce or candy), and colas and other sweetened soft drinks.

6.14: Additional Solutions:

Losing weight after the age of 50 can be more challenging, but it is not impossible. While the aging process can affect our metabolism and hormonal balance, it doesn't mean we have to accept weight gain as inevitable. Even after the age of 50, it is still feasible to reach and maintain a healthy weight by a mix of nutritious food, regular physical exercise, and lifestyle changes. It's critical to focus on making long-term adjustments to your eating habits, such as choosing nutrient-dense meals, reducing portion sizes, and avoiding excessive sugary and processed food intake. Regular physical activity, including both cardiovascular and strength training, can assist enhance metabolism, preserve muscle mass, and help with weight loss attempts. Additionally, managing stress levels, getting enough sleep, and staying hydrated are all important factors in maintaining a healthy weight. Weight reduction may take longer and involve more work as we age, but it is possible to reach and maintain a healthy weight at any age with dedication and a balanced approach.

6.14.1: Supplements?

What's good? You don't need most vitamins. It's also time to think bigger, like giving your plate the best mix of foods.

"People often ask about different supplements, but we want them to focus on eating in a balanced way," says Emily Blake, a registered dietitian at Brigham and Women's Hospital, which is connected to Harvard. "Quick fixes are often promoted as a gateway to health, when more sustainable changes are what's going to move the needle."

D3 from food.

Vitamin D deficiency is very common as we age because not many things naturally contain a lot of it. It might be easier to get enough sun in the summer for our skin to make vitamin D, but we need to weigh that benefit against the risk of skin cancer. Fatigue, bone pain, mood swings, muscle aches, and weakness are all signs of insufficiency.

Milk and cereals that have been enhanced with vitamin D, soy milk, mushrooms, canned tuna, shrimp, and salmon are all good sources of vitamin D. people up to age 70 should get 600 IU of vitamin D every day, and people 71 and older should get 800 IU. A daily 1,000-IU vitamin D supplement is enough to meet this need.

Iron.

Red blood cells move oxygen around the body and need enough iron to work properly. But being pregnant or having heavy periods can wear us down and leave us wanting. Plant-based diets, which are becoming more popular, can also work because iron is easier for our bodies to receive from animal sources than from plant-based sources.

You might feel cold, tired, or short of breath if you don't have enough iron in your body. You might get headaches more often. Meat and fish usually have a lot of iron. Beans, lentils, grains, spinach, and cereals that have been fortified are plant-based sources of iron. Over-50-year-old women need 8 mg of iron every day, while younger women need 18 mg.

The vitamin B12.

B12 is important for nerve signals and making red blood cells, but as we age, our bodies become less good at absorbing it. Since plants don't have the vitamin, vegans and vegetarians are also more likely to be deficient.

Anemia can make you tired, and a lack of B12 can make your hands, legs, and feet feel numb. You may also have trouble walking and keeping your balance. The memory can also get worse. Fish, chicken, milk, and cheese are all good sources of vitamin B12. Try enriched nondairy milks and cereals if you'd rather eat plant-based foods. Every day, adults need 2.4 micrograms of B12.

Calcium is important.

Most of us know that calcium helps our bones stay strong. It also helps our muscles and nerves work properly and keeps our heartbeat steady. As estrogen levels drop, our bodies become less able to absorb calcium. People who don't eat dairy can make the risk even higher.

Cow's milk, soy or almond milks that have been fortified, yogurt, cheese, fortified cereals, and dark green veggies like broccoli and kale are all good sources of calcium. Every day, most people need 1,000 mg, but women over 50 need 1,200 mg.

6.14.2: Some health issues to be addressed
Muscles and bones break down faster when they aren't used enough, and being weak can make you lazy, which is the last thing your body needs to get strong. Getting in shape can help, though. To keep your muscles working and your bones strong, do weight-bearing activities like walking and strength training. Also, nutrition is very important. Calcium can be found in dairy, almonds, and vegetables, so make sure you get enough of it in your food. Some dairy alternatives are fortified oat or coconut milk, leafy veggies like bok choy, beans, lentils, and seeds like chia and sesame. Another option is to eat nuts or dairy-free foods. To get calcium into the bones, you need vitamin D, which you can get from tuna, sardines, egg yolks, and foods that have been added to them. Sunlight is another way for the skin to get vitamin D. Some people, especially those who live in the Northeast and have darker melanin, may need to take supplements. Studies show that this type of skin gets less vitamin D from the sun

because melanin in the skin stops the process of making it. Also, more people of color test negative for vitamin D deficiency, but more of them also test positive for better bone mineral density than white people. The cause? The amount of vitamin D-binding protein in their bodies is smaller, but their bodies still let the same amount of the nutrient be used. So, a vitamin D level test can help make things clear.

If you have any signs, like soft or weak bones, aches in your lower back, pelvis, hips, legs, or ribs, or if your muscles aren't as toned or you have trouble walking, your healthcare team can tell if you would benefit from a supplement and what dose you should take.

7.0: Final decision - The Right one for Me?

With so many options overwhelming us, it will be prudent for us to give a concrete solution for effective weight loss objective. However, the weight loss process is so complicated that it will be almost impossible for anyone to provide that coveted answer. Hence, we are going to share some of the best strategies - from experts' ends to achieve the goal.

7.1: Expert View One:

Fundamentals of Weight Loss for Women Over 50:

A particularly difficult concept to grasp in regards to weight loss, particularly for women over the age of 50, is the following:

It is advised that we consume approximately 2000 calories per day, as this is roughly the number of calories our bodies expend in a 24-hour period simply by remaining sedentary.

Calorie consumption occurs even in the absence of physical activity; however, as you age, the daily caloric expenditure varies.

Studies indicate that as we age, our bodies use fewer calories, regardless of exercise, which means that in order to lose weight, we must increase our physical activity. Furthermore, women require fewer calories than men, which creates an even greater challenge.

According to the American Council on Exercise, for each ten years of age that passes, women expend 150 fewer calories per day. Thus, while a physically robust 20-year-old woman may expend 2000 calories on a daily basis, an individual aged 50 burns only 1,550 calories, and this is prior to any dietary or activity modifications.

Obviously, these are approximations, but the point remains clear: your body simply no longer burns as many calories naturally as it once did; any calories that remain are typically stored as fat.

Therefore, when discussing weight loss for women over the age of 50, it is important to recognize that adjustments that account for this difference in calorie expenditure are necessary for weight maintenance or loss.

Weight Loss for Women Over the Age of 50 - Making More Intelligent Decisions:

When considering this matter exclusively in terms of calories, there are only two viable approaches to resolve the situation: reduce caloric intake or increase expenditure.

Obviously, the most effective way to lose weight is to combine exercise and diet. Following a lifetime of poor choices, this may seem like an overwhelming transition for women over the age of 50 who have never before exercised or dieted. However, it does not have to be this way.

Ingesting less necessitates making more informed dietary choices by keeping in mind one's objectives and the difficulties associated with weight loss after the age of 50. From a dietary standpoint, it may resemble the following:

• A reduced number of munchies;

• An improved selection of snacks;

• A decrease in sugar intake;

• An increased consumption of fruits and vegetables in lieu of processed foods.

• Basic portion management

These are a few recommendations that may assist you in consuming fewer calories on the whole.

Rather than advocating for an extreme or restrictive diet, the focus should be on making more rational decisions.

However, seeing results is unlikely if you do not approach this issue from two different directions: exercise and diet. Diet is the first front, and the second is exercise.

Weight Loss—Even a modest increase in activity can assist women over 50 in losing weight.

Weight loss—Diet is frequently the cause of significant weight gain in women over the age of 50, but physical activity should not be disregarded.

Active living increases caloric expenditure, which aids in maintaining body weight below the individual limit—the threshold at which surplus calories are stored as adipose tissue.

Although some individuals become anxious at the mere mention of exercise, there is no need for alarm! Triathlon training, CrossFit, or significant weightlifting are probably unnecessary to achieve noticeable progress.

Simplify matters further; any one or a combination of the following would facilitate increased daily caloric expenditure and bring about progress towards weight loss:

• Increasing the distance or speed of evening walks gradually

• Swimming or water-walking a few times per week

• Bicycling or walking to work

• Bicycle rides around the neighborhood

• Enrolling in a novices' yoga class

• Becoming a member of the beginners' group at a local running club

There are quite a few hundred ways to incorporate some form of physical activity into one's daily routine.

It is crucial to exercise moderation, as excessive physical activity can have an impact on hormone levels.

Maintain a light and entertaining tone instead. Find something enjoyable to do, or at the very least, engage in an activity that allows you to listen to your preferred podcast, audiobook, or music, or even watch Netflix or television.

In the context of weight loss, it is particularly imperative for women aged 50 and above to identify a consistent activity. It can be particularly difficult to maintain changes that are extreme or disagreeable, and as one ages, it becomes increasingly difficult to initiate any changes. Already, losing weight after the age of 50 is difficult enough. It need not be made worse than it already is.

7.2: Expert View Two:

Changing one's lifestyle significantly can be difficult, particularly as one ages. In order to increase your NEAT (Non-Exercise Activity Thermogenesis) intake and build muscle, it may be beneficial to develop a consistent exercise regimen or weight loss strategy.

Choose one or two enjoyable exercises that target muscle development, as well as several varied methods to incorporate more physical activity, and construct a regimen around those components. Additionally, it is advisable to contemplate the frequency of each exercise, such as the number of times per week that strength training will be performed. This can assist you in maintaining motivation and provide you with attainable objectives to strive for.

Decrease Stress

Sadly, every individual must contend with tension on a daily schedule. However, the nature of tension may manifest itself differently in individuals.

Inflammation can result from chronic stress, and inflammation can contribute to weight gain, particularly with advancing age. Consequently, in addition to enhancing one's overall health, tension reduction may also facilitate weight loss.

After identifying the source of tension in one's life, several strategies to mitigate it can be generated. Simply articulating your requirements might suffice. Additional methods include journaling, meditating, sleeping enough, and basking in the sun.

Exclude Potential Conditions Like Hypothyroidism

As previously stated, age increases the prevalence of certain conditions, including subclinical hypothyroidism, a risk factor for weight gain. Should you experience unforeseen fluctuations in your body composition, it might be prudent to consult your physician or other healthcare professional about this.

A consultation with your physician can assist in the exclusion of latent or unidentified factors that could be implicated in your weight gain.

7.3: Expert View Three:

Researchers have found a link between bad belly fat and more inflammation, heart disease, and diabetes. But you can avoid this by eating well and working out to keep your weight in check, which is especially important as you get older. The Physical Activity Guidelines for Americans say that you should be active for 30 minutes most days, and on two days you should do strength training. It's best to be active at least three times a week. You should also do muscle-strengthening exercises like sit-ups or moving weights at least twice a week. A good way to improve your balance is to do yoga, Tai Chi, or balance poses like Tree Pose (standing on one foot).

For a healthy heart, eat a lot of fruits, veggies, and whole grains. It looks like estrogen helps keep the walls of arteries open and may even out the amount of good and bad cholesterol in the body. Blood veins get stiffer as we age, which makes the heart work harder. This makes high blood pressure worse. High blood pressure makes you more likely to get heart disease or a stroke because it hurts the walls of your arteries and lets plaque buildup, which makes the arteries narrow. To keep blood pressure low, you can do moderate exercise, get 7-8 hours of sleep every night, and learn how to deal with worry.

If you want to lower your chance of getting breast cancer, you should keep a healthy weight, work out regularly, drink less alcohol, and if you take hormone replacement therapy, do not do it for more than five years. Mammograms should be done regularly on women over 50. You might want to start getting mammograms earlier if you are younger and have a history of breast cancer in your family. At least once a month, all women, no matter what age, should check their breasts at home. Pay close attention to any lumps you feel, especially if they are hard and have an odd shape. Also, pay attention to any lumps that weren't there before. Check for changes in the skin's texture, like puckering, dimpling, indentations, or nipples that have turned inward. Also, look for changes in the skin's tone, especially around the areola.

Simple Kegel movements can help keep your pelvic floor strong. If your bladder is empty, squeeze as if you were holding your pee for 5 to 10 seconds. Then let go. Do five to ten of these several times a day. It can also help to stay away from caffeine, booze, sodas, and foods that are very acidic.

Eating a lot of acidic foods can irritate the walls of the bladder and make pelvic floor problems worse.

Taking Care of Your Skin as It Gets Older

Eating well, getting enough good sleep, drinking lots of water, and not smoking are all important for healthy, glowing skin at any age, but they become even more important as you get older. You can get rid of lines naturally by doing things like exfoliating and putting on a retinol night cream. But staying out of the sun is the most important thing you can do. You might also want to switch from hot showers to warm showers because hot showers dry out the skin. Also, smoking can make lines show up, so you might want to give up.

No matter what age you are or how bad your hair is, you can make it healthier by staying away from strong chemicals and being gentle with it.

7.4: Expert View Four:

Consider including these delectable alternatives into your diet in order to mitigate bone resorption and reduce the risk of experiencing fractures.

Adhering to a diverse dietary regimen may entail consuming certain foods just for enjoyment purposes, while others are consumed for their functional benefits. Prunes are commonly classified in the latter category, being generally recognized as a dietary aid for maintaining regular bowel movements. However, recent study indicates that these dehydrated plums possess multiple benefits, extending beyond their initial reputation, by enhancing both digestive function and bone density.

The findings of the research, which was published in the October 2022 edition of The American Journal of Clinical Nutrition, indicate that the regular consumption of five or six prunes per day by postmenopausal women can contribute to the maintenance of bone mineral density in the hip region, potentially reducing the risk of bone fractures. The researchers conducted a year-long study including 235 elderly women, during which they observed that the regular consumption of a small quantity of prunes appeared to reduce the presence of inflammatory substances that are known to contribute to the degradation of bone tissue.

Following the onset of menopause, women often experience a rapid decline in bone density, rendering them significantly more susceptible to the development of osteoporosis, a condition characterized by weakened bones. This phenomenon is observed to a greater extent in women compared to males. Approximately 75% of hip fractures occur in females, and this particular injury significantly heightens the likelihood of experiencing a decline in autonomy and a shortened lifespan. Furthermore, as per the National Institutes of Health, it has been reported that a significant proportion, specifically 50%, of women aged 50 and beyond are expected to experience fractures in their hip, wrist, or spine at some point in their lifespan.

According to Dr. Harold Rosen, the director of the Osteoporosis Prevention and Treatment Center at Harvard-affiliated Beth Israel Deaconess Medical Center, the potential efficacy of prunes in promoting bone health may not be substantial. However, considering their additional advantages, the threshold for recommending their consumption would be relatively low.

However, prunes are not the only surprising item that has advantages for bone health.

The term "dynamic duo" refers to a pair of individuals who work together in a highly effective and synergistic manner.

In contrast to prunes, the majority of food and beverage options that are recognized for their ability to enhance bone health achieve this through the inclusion of calcium, a significant constituent of bones. The optimal efficacy of the mineral is observed when it is combined with vitamin D, since the latter facilitates the absorption of calcium within the body.

The process of bone remodeling involves the ongoing breakdown and subsequent rebuilding of bone tissue, which is considered a normal physiological occurrence. The bones facilitate the release of stored calcium into the bloodstream, which serves several physiological activities such as blood clotting and muscle contractions. To maintain an adequate calcium supply, we replace it through dietary intake.

The attainment of peak bone mass typically occurs at approximately 30 years of age, after which it remains rather stable for a duration of almost two decades. However, postmenopausal women experience a higher rate of bone loss that surpasses the rate of bone regeneration in their bodies. The process of aging can induce the body to extract calcium from bones.

It is widely recognized that primary sources of calcium encompass dairy items, such as milk, yogurt, and cheese, as well as dark leafy greens, including collards, kale, Swiss chard, and broccoli. Minerals are frequently added to breakfast cereals and fruit juices for fortification purposes.

However, it is possible that you are not cognizant of these alternative food sources that provide a substantial amount of calcium.

Dried figs are a type of fruit that has undergone a dehydration process, resulting in a shriveled and preserved form. Two figs typically contain approximately 65 milligrams (mg) of calcium. Similar to prunes (and potentially even more delectable than their relative), figs have the ability to be thinly cut and added to oatmeal or included into smoothies. In addition, they exhibit excellent compatibility when combined with cheese, and can even serve as a topping for pizzas.

Canned salmon is a type of preserved fish that has been cooked, deboned, and packaged in a can for long-term storage. The calcium content in a serving size of 3 ounces is 180 mg. According to Dr. Rosen, canned salmon contains a significant amount of minerals due to the presence of small, unnoticeable bones. He further asserts that a typical salmon filet has a mere 36 mg of calcium, a quantity that he does not consider to be a significant supply. One can easily combine canned salmon with mayonnaise to create a sandwich spread, similar to the method used with tuna, or alternatively, blend it to produce a dip.

What about plant-based milk alternatives? Cow's milk is commonly regarded as a reliable and substantial source of dietary calcium, and this perception is well-founded. However, plant-based milk alternatives such as almond, rice, or soy milk are commonly fortified in order to achieve a calcium content comparable to that of traditional dairy milk. An 8-ounce quantity typically has a range of 350 to 400 milligrams. It is advisable to scrutinize product labels and exercise caution regarding the presence of added sugars in plant-based milk alternatives.

Tofu, a soy-based food product, is a popular dietary staple in many cultures. The soy-based staple of Asian gastronomy has 430 mg of calcium per 4-ounce meal, with calcium-fortified variations frequently containing twice that quantity. Soy foods, such as edamame, are typically characterized by a high calcium content, which is significant for bone health. Additionally, they serve as a crucial source of protein, which also contributes to maintaining optimal bone health.

What about almonds and almond butter? Almonds are widely recognized for their cardiovascular advantages, making them highly appealing despite their high caloric content. The nuts alone contain 190 mg of calcium in a half-cup serving, but 2 tablespoons of almond butter provide 111 mg of calcium.

Canned white beans. Each cup of legumes, including navy, cannellini, great northern, and lima beans, contains approximately 190 mg of calcium, making them a valuable addition to soups and stews. According to Dr. Rosen, beans are a valuable source of protein.

7.5: Expert View Five:
Addressing deficiencies

Incorporating lesser-known sources of calcium into one's dietary intake might augment the advantages for bone health, beyond the benefits derived from commonly consumed staples like dairy products and dark leafy greens. What is the recommended daily intake of calcium? According to the guidelines set forth by the National Academy of Medicine, it is recommended that women aged 50 and below has a daily calcium intake of 1,000 mg, while women aged 51 and above should aim for a daily calcium intake of 1,200 mg. In order to optimize its efficacy, it is advisable to supplement calcium consumption with a daily intake of 800 international units (IU) of vitamin D, especially in regions with limited access to natural sunlight.

It is advisable to consult product labels in order to determine the precise quantities of calcium and vitamin D that are typically obtained from one's daily dietary intake. The individual is advised to first evaluate one's nutritional status. After calculating the sum of the figures, one can compensate for the disparity between the suggested and real quantities by utilizing dietary supplements.

However, it is important to exercise moderation and avoid excessive behavior. There is compelling data indicating that the consumption of calcium-vitamin D combination supplements by women is associated with an increased susceptibility to the development of kidney stones. According to Dr. Rosen, individuals have historically strived to increase their daily calcium consumption; nevertheless, he expresses skepticism regarding the merits of this approach.

Additionally, it is advisable to use caution when considering various supplementary products that purport to have advantages for bone health. The utilization of the heavy metal strontium is frequently promoted for this specific purpose. However, scientific investigations have revealed that its effects are limited to enhancing the visual appearance of bone density on imaging scans.

In order to effectively enhance bone strength while minimizing the risk of injury, it is advisable to engage in low-impact exercise.

Consuming foods that are abundant in calcium and vitamin D significantly contributes to the preservation of optimal bone health. However, engaging in physical exercise, particularly activities that involve exerting one's own body weight in opposition to gravity, also serves to boost bone strength and promote its maintenance.

According to Dr. Harold Rosen, director of the Osteoporosis Prevention and Treatment Center at Beth Israel Deaconess Medical Center, older adults who are at a greater risk of developing osteoporosis, a condition characterized by the weakening of bones, should likely disregard popular recommendations promoting jump training or high-impact activities that involve repetitive pounding on the ground.

Dr. Rosen expresses a disapproval towards the concept of pounding. Although there is a certain degree of logic to this perspective, it is important to acknowledge that it also has the potential to result in physical harm. Many elderly individuals commonly experience shoulder or knee issues, which may be exacerbated by engaging in activities that place excessive stress on their skeletal structures.

According to the speaker, incorporating low-impact alternatives into one's routine can effectively maintain bone strength in a safer manner. The physical activities that fall under this category encompass walking briskly outdoors or on a treadmill, engaging in stair climbing using a machine, participating in low-impact aerobics, and utilizing elliptical training machines.

7.6: Expert View Six:

Identify the presence of osteoporosis prior to experiencing a bone fracture

Osteoporosis, a medical condition characterized by the weakening and fragility of bones, affects a significantly higher number of elderly women compared to males, with a ratio of four to one. This discrepancy can be attributed, at least in part, to the decline of estrogen levels following menopause, which plays a role in safeguarding bone health. However, it is worth noting that as individuals age, there is a possibility of experiencing a decrease in height or the development of a slightly bent posture, which may serve as indications of the presence of osteoporosis. Nevertheless, it is important to acknowledge that osteoporosis often remains asymptomatic until a bone fracture occurs.

However, bone density testing can serve as a means to prevent such a distressing situation. The DEXA scan, a form of x-ray technology, is utilized to assess the mineral density of bones, particularly calcium and other minerals. Osteoporosis can be detected prior to the occurrence of a potentially hazardous fracture. The DEXA technique has the capability to forecast an individual's susceptibility to a forthcoming bone fracture, as well as evaluate the efficacy of osteoporosis therapy.

It is advised that bone density testing be conducted for women aged 65 and above, with subsequent testing occurring biennially. In the age range of 50 to 64, it is recommended that women with specific risk factors for osteoporosis, such as low body weight, previous fractures, a parental history of hip fracture, presence of diseases associated with bone loss, or usage of medications known to cause bone thinning, should also initiate regular screening.

What is the procedure for conducting DEXA scanning? During a 15-minute duration, the individual will assume a supine position on a cushioned table. During the examination, a single x-ray device will traverse across the region including the hips and lower spine, while a separate x-ray device will travel beneath same region. Similar to other x-ray examinations, it will be necessary for you to maintain immobility and suspend respiration during specific intervals.

The examination will yield two scores. A comparison is made between an individual's bone density and that of a healthy young adult. The second method involves comparing it to others of similar age, gender, and ethnic origin. There is a positive correlation between an individual's score and the density of their bones. Although existing standards assist healthcare professionals in making treatment decisions for individuals with poor bone density, additional study is required to ascertain the accuracy of ethnicity-related criteria.

7.7: Expert View Seven:
Implementing fuel

There are numerous methods for burning retained excess fat. The first is to decrease your caloric consumption. When the body's caloric intake falls below its requirements', stored fat is converted into usable energy for propulsion purposes. As a consequence, adipose cells diminish in size and weight loss ensues.

Due to the fact that carbohydrates are the body's principal source of calories, low-carb regimens adhere to this strategy. According to research, while low-carb regimens may aid in initiating weight loss, the effect may diminish within six months to a year. "Part of the problem is that low-carb diets are tough to maintain for long periods," according to Dr. Apovian.

Many nutritionists advocate for a well-rounded, health-promoting diet that comprises sufficient quantities of protein, carbohydrates, and lipids, in addition to vital vitamins and minerals. "A low-carb diet can help in the short term, but if you don't adjust your overall eating habits, you can gain it all back," according to Dr. Apovian.

Exercise is another method for burning fat and reducing fat cell size. Aerobic exercise of a moderate intensity, such as brisk strolling, cycling, and swimming, can compel the body to utilize fat reserves as an energy source. (Recommendations call for a minimum of 150 minutes of moderate-intensity exercise per week.) The rate at which your body consumes fat, however, is dependent on your body mass and exercise intensity.

By increasing muscle mass, resistance (weight) training can also assist older men in losing excess fat that has been retained. "Men naturally lose muscle mass as they age, and increasing muscle can make their body burn more calories," according to Dr. Apovian.

An online analysis published by Sports Medicine on September 21, 2021, discovered that individuals who performed resistance training for 45 to 60 minutes, twice to three times per week, over the course of five months experienced a reduction in visceral fat as well as total body fat.

However, relying solely on exercise is insufficient for weight loss. Additionally, you must decrease your caloric consumption, advises Dr. Apovian. "And to help keep it off, you need to do resistance training at least two to three times per week."

7.8: Expert View Eight:
Strategies for mitigating weight increase during midlife

According to medical professionals, menopausal hormone therapy may offer potential benefits for women experiencing midlife weight gains. This therapeutic approach involves the administration of a combination of estrogen and progesterone to alleviate the symptoms associated with menopause, including but not limited to hot flashes.

An expert posits that extant evidence indicates the potential of hormone therapy to ameliorate the adipose redistribution occurring in the abdominal region during the menopausal phase. Additionally, it has the potential to mitigate sleep disturbances and mental disorders that may have an indirect influence on the accumulation of body weight.

Nevertheless, medical professionals assert that hormone therapy in itself will not be enough for women in effectively managing their weight gain around midlife. It is advisable for women to incorporate strength or resistance training into their exercise routines in order to mitigate the effects of muscle loss.

According to Sylvia Gonsahn-Bollie, a physician based in Silver Spring, Maryland, many individuals possess a strong affinity for cardiovascular exercises. However, it is advisable to strive for a balanced routine with equal proportions of cardiovascular activities and resistance training. Specifically, it is recommended that individuals engage in physical activity for a minimum of 150 minutes each week in order to achieve weight loss and sustain it. However, it is worth mentioning that a majority of individuals may require a higher range of 300 to 420 minutes.

According to Gonsahn-Bollie, effective stress management is crucial due to its potential to induce chronic stress, hence elevating cortisol levels. This hormonal response can subsequently lead to heightened insulin resistance, posing challenges in weight loss endeavors.

In addition to engaging in physical activity and implementing stress management techniques, dietary modifications can also contribute to facilitating weight management among women. It is advisable for women to increase their consumption of protein and fiber while concurrently decreasing their intake of sugar.

In accordance with the perspective of Ekta Kapoor, an esteemed associate professor of medicine at Mayo Clinic in Minnesota, it is advisable for women below the age of 40 to strive for a state of perimenopause while maintaining a healthy body weight, a determination that may be facilitated by a medical professional. For women endeavoring to achieve weight loss amid the present circumstances, it is advised to establish pragmatic expectations, as the process may out to be more challenging than initially anticipated.

7.9: Expert View Nine:

Do I need to consume half as much to lose weight? If not, what is a reasonable daily calorie intake? Assuming you are as active as you were at age 20, you require 200 fewer calories per day at 50. You require 400–500 fewer calories after 60. Aim for about 2,000 calories per day if you're moderately active up to the age of 50. You should cut back to 1,800 calories after 50.

Must I exercise twice as hard? If no, how frequently? Exercise intensifiers falsely believe they are burning more calories than they actually are. Exercise alone will not result in significant weight loss, despite common assumption, and you cannot exercise off a poor diet, no matter how intense your workouts are. Moreover, you run the risk of overeating if you exercise twice as hard. Therefore, it is not advised doing twice as much exercise in order to eat twice as much. Cutting calories and engaging in moderate physical activity for thirty to sixty minutes each day are advised.

How can my metabolism be increased? Three approaches exist:

• Exercise for strength. It used to be all cardio, cardio, and more cardio. However, gaining muscle mass speeds up your metabolism by enabling you to burn more calories while at rest. As you age, your muscular mass decreases. Consume breakfast. Your body gets fuel from it for the entire day. You become hungrier later if you skip breakfast. Eating a hearty breakfast, a moderate lunch, and a light dinner is ideal.

• Consume more lean protein-rich foods, such as tofu, poultry, fish, and eggs. This gives you energy for the day and aids in the growth of muscle, which raises metabolism.

Are there any particular meals that help speed up metabolism? According to certain research, meals high in capsaicin, which is present in chili peppers, can speed up metabolism. Sip a lot of water. Additionally, green tea might increase metabolism.

Are there any particular foods I should never consume? No food should ever be avoided. You shouldn't consider yourself to be being deprived. It goes without saying that you shouldn't frequently consume alcohol, fried food, or highly processed meals. Just consume little amounts of it.

Food cravings are exacerbated by processed meals like refined sugar and white flour, which also alter blood sugar levels. Take a day off if you eat clean—that is, whole, unprocessed foods—six days a week. Simply resume eating healthily the following day.

Which are some useful resources? Portion control is an important lesson that Weight Watchers teaches, which is why it is appreciated. You may also log what you eat with the free food journal feature of the My Fitness Pal app. It makes you more aware of what you're eating and holds you accountable. Activity trackers like Fitbits also assist in increasing your step count. Does my metabolism change when I sleep? Sleep plays a critical role in our weight. According to studies, those who don't get enough sleep tend to eat more calories and gain weight. Hormonal dysregulation brought on by sleep deprivation results in food cravings. Everyone has to get into bed sooner.

Does metabolism depend on heredity? Everything is impacted by heredity. A portion of a person's quick metabolism is inherited. Then there are those who gain weight when they glance sideways at a doughnut. It's annoying that some people will drop weight more quickly. All you have is what you have to work with. When you're trying so hard to lose weight and it's hardly coming off, it can be difficult to keep your motivation up. Maintain a nutritious lifestyle and engage in regular exercise, and the weight will drop off.

Do some drugs cause a slowdown in metabolism? Numerous drugs, such as steroids, antidepressants, diabetic meds, and anti-seizure medications, might result in weight gain. They may increase fluid retention, slow down metabolism, and increase hunger, encouraging you to eat more. If a patient claims, "I just keep gaining weight, and I'm eating well and exercising," they ought to discuss their medications with their doctors. Consult your doctor to see whether your medications could be contributing to your weight gain before stopping them suddenly.

7.10: Expert View Ten

Strategies to Prevent Age-Related Weight Gain

Even while dealing with weight gain that comes with becoming older can be challenging, once you turn 50, you can take proactive measures to prevent it. If you're experiencing weight gain as a result of aging, you might want to try the useful advice below.

1.   Maintaining proper hydration

Keeping yourself properly hydrated is essential for managing your weight, especially as you become older. A study on the advantages of drinking water was done on an older adult population. The researchers found that when older persons followed a low-calorie diet, drinking two cups of water prior to meals appeared to help them lose more weight. This may be explained by the fact that drinking enough water helps control hunger and heighten sensations of fullness. While staying hydrated is crucial, it's best to focus on drinking water and low-sugar drinks like coconut water.

2.   Boost your intake of protein and Put on Muscle.

You can prevent sarcopenia and maintain more muscle mass by eating more protein. Experts advise persons over 65, whether inactive or active, to consume between 1.2 and 2.0

grams of protein per kilogram of body weight. Protein is an essential component of a healthy diet.

On the other hand, elderly persons with chronic conditions or those recuperating from illnesses or injuries could find it advantageous to consume a higher protein intake of 1.6 to 2.5 grams per kilogram of bodyweight.

Getting enough protein in your diet can help you maintain more muscle mass and raise your resting metabolic rate. The building blocks for hormones like T3, T4, insulin, and leptin—all of which tend to decline with age—can be obtained by increasing your protein intake.

Increasing your muscular mass can help sustain your body as it ages and increase your metabolism. It can also support healthy insulin levels and fat burning. It is advised that you include strength or resistance training in your workout regimen to efficiently build muscle. Working with a personal trainer can help you create a personalized strategy based on your unique health needs if you're new to the gym.

If weight training isn't your thing, you might want to try something like jazzercise, which blends aerobic and low weight training. Finding a fun sport that supports your muscle-building objectives is essential, as is making regular exercise a weekly priority.

3.   Boost Your Day's Non-Exercise Activity Thermogenesis (NEAT)

Increasing your daily non-exercise activity thermogenesis (NEAT) can help you lose weight and improve your general health. The calories burnt via regular physical activity that isn't a part of a regimented workout program are referred to as NEAT.

Surprisingly, NEAT exercises can increase your metabolic rate and account for 15 to 30 percent of your daily caloric expenditure. This is especially beneficial when it comes to preventing age-related weight gain. Walking, doing chores around the house, gardening, and even simple hobbies like folding clothes are examples of NEAT activities. You may boost your weight reduction efforts and improve your calorie burn by raising your NEAT.

7.11: Expert View Eleven:

7 Science-Backed Ways to Battle the Bulge at Midlife and Beyond

There are specific, effective tactics you can deploy to retake control of your weight.

1. Prioritize Nutritious Foods

Griebeler, an expert.   recommends cutting down on processed foods like fast food and added sugar and upping your diet of fruits and vegetables. Lustgarten, another expert, recommends focusing on high-fiber whole foods including vegetables, beans, nuts, whole grains, and fruit. "It will make it easier to monitor calories. She notes that these foods are large in volume because they fill up more of the stomach yet contribute less calories overall.

2. Reduce Your Serving Sizes

It takes time to adjust your diet to meet your body's reduced caloric needs. Griebeler recommends reducing your caloric intake by 100–200 calories daily at first. One approach to keep track of what you eat is to use a calorie tracking app. It's amazing how much of a difference even a minor adjustment can make.

3. Keep Yourself Hydrated

It's simple to confuse thirst with hunger. A review of multiple animal studies published in June 2016 in Frontiers in Nutrition reveals that drinking water (instead of calorie-rich beverages like sodas, fancy coffee drinks, and fruit juices) can increase metabolic rate and the rate at which fat is broken down.

4. Identify Methods for Controlling Stress

According to Griebeler, stress causes binge eating in many people. Take whatever steps you need to unwind, be it a yoga session twice a week or several daily five-minute meditations.

5: Workout Your Larger Muscle Groups

That earlier-mentioned decrease in muscular mass? Strength training should be part of your fitness routine as a means of self-defense. "You want to preserve muscle mass as much as possible," adds Griebeler. Gaining muscle improves your metabolism and makes you more active due to enhanced coordination and stamina. The Go4Life program from the National Institute on Aging is a great way to get started with simple at-home strengthening exercises.

6. You Should Be More Active

Try to add a half hour a day of aerobic exercise — which is anything that gets your heart rate up, such as jogging, walking, bicycling, or swimming, recommends Lustgarten. Can't find a way to free up 30 minutes at once? You can break up the time by taking three 10-minute walks at different times throughout the day. It's true that "short bursts of activity have a cumulative effect and count toward a daily exercise goal," as she puts it.

7. Get Some Restful Sleep

You won't be as active during the day and thus won't burn as many calories if you don't feel motivated when you wake up. The recommended amount of sleep per night, according to Primack, is between seven and nine hours.

1. Maintaining Strong Bones and Heart Health Through Exercise and Nutrition

Vulnerable bones and joints: as reaching postmenopause time to time triggers calcium deficiency leading to feebler frames, a blend of diet ensuring nutrition and fair amount of exercise can ensure a graceful living for a woman in her 50s.

An approach to boosting or at least preserving your brain power - as well as retention power - is to commit yourself to a Mediterranean diet: containing healthy fats like olive and canola oils, veggies, whole grains, and fruits.

More fat around the middle does more than just make buttoning jeans difficult. According to studies, visceral adipose tissue, or belly fat, is also bad for your health.

 Fix: Exercises for the abdomen won't eliminate belly fat on their own. Instead, concentrate on losing weight overall by adopting a healthier lifestyle. Cutting back on alcohol or dining no later than six o'clock in the evening are easy ways to reduce your daily calorie intake. Next, figure out how to increase your level of exercise. Experts suggest aiming for an hour of activity every day, but even a slight increase makes an effect.

2. Have a grip on your alcohol consumption

As you age, your body metabolizes alcohol more slowly while our muscle mass decreases, leaving less muscle tissue available to assimilate alcohol.

Try a mocktail as a remedy. You can have a great after-dinner drink without drinking alcohol, thanks to the increasing variety of booze-free beverages available on the market. If you do decide to drink, make sure you abide by the U.S. Dietary Guidelines, which recommend that women limit their daily alcohol intake to one standard drink. In general, that equals 1.5 ounces of spirits, 5 ounces of wine, or 12 ounces of beer.

3. You may not be aware of the increased risk of heart disease.

The solution: Use a calculator to calculate your own risk of a cardiovascular incident within the next ten years, or ask your healthcare physician to do so. Next, concentrate on reducing hazards that you can manage by changing to a healthy way of living. Increasing your daily physical activity will yield the greatest returns. In terms of food, steer clear of saturated fat and consume more plants.

4. Sexual relations could become awkward

Low hormone levels after menopause cause the vaginal walls to thin and dry, which can cause discomfort, painful sex, and a decrease in desire

The solution: Over-the-counter moisturizers and lubricants work wonders for certain ladies. If not, discuss other forms of hormone therapy with your physician. Vaginal estrogen cream "can build back up the lining of the vagina, which helps with lubrication and to maintain elasticity" and is safe for the majority of women.

5. Your sleeping habits alter

If you've experienced menopause, you may be familiar with how a hot flash may startle you out of a deep sleep and leave you drenched in perspiration.

The solution: Sleep hygiene might help you achieve a restful night's sleep, according to research. Every night, try to go to bed and wake up at about the same time. Make sure your bedroom is as dark as you can. And at night, lower the thermostat to 65 to 67 degrees Fahrenheit. Daily exercise and exposure to bright light are also crucial.

6. You develop more fragile bones

Everyone begins to lose some bone density around the age of 50.

The solution: Weight-bearing exercises that improve bone include strength training, walking, hiking, climbing stairs, tennis, and dancing. According to experts, "it shifts the formative structures inside the bone, telling the bones to stay strong." Make sure you consume adequate calcium and vitamin D at the same time, either through food or supplements. Aim for at least 600 IU of vitamin D and 1,200 mg of calcium every day.

Additionally, you need to focus on the following advices.

• Consider the long term rather than passing trends.

"You should avoid following a diet that limits your food options," experts suggest. Make sustaining healthy food choices instead. Limit your intake of sweets and alcohol, as well as your carbohydrates.

• Concentrate on wholesome protein sources.

According to an expert, "protein keeps you fuller for longer and helps you avoid blood sugar spikes that come from all-carbohydrate meals." "If you want oatmeal for breakfast, for instance, you may up the protein content by adding some nuts or peanut butter."

• Be mindful while you eat.

"Aim to eat through by 8 p.m.," an expert advises. "The ideal window of time between your last meal of the day and bedtime is three hours or more."

• Exert yourself.

"Every day, ideally for at least 30 minutes, engage in physical activity that elevates your heart rate," advises the expert. "That can be anything you enjoy doing, like biking, swimming, jogging, walking, or working out to YouTube videos."

• **Gain or maintain muscle mass.**

As we age, we tend to lose muscle mass because, at rest, muscle consumes more calories than fat. You should include strengthening exercises in your program at least two days a week, advises the expert.

7.13: Expert View Thirteen:

It can be more difficult for many people to maintain a healthy weight or reduce excess body fat as they age. A sedentary lifestyle, poor dietary choices, unhealthy habits, and changes in metabolism can all lead to weight increase after the age of fifty. However, regardless of your athletic capabilities or medical diagnoses, you can lose weight at any age with a few easy tweaks. The top 20 methods for weight loss after 50 are listed here.

1. Develop a passion for strength training

While aerobic exercise is often the focus when it comes to weight loss, strength training is just as vital, particularly for older folks. A condition known as sarcopenia causes your muscle mass to decrease as you age. Your metabolism may slow down due to this loss of muscle mass, which starts to happen around the age of 50 and could result in weight gain.

You lose roughly 1% to 2% of your muscle mass and 1.5% to 5% of your muscle strength year after the age of 50. For this reason, include muscle-building workouts in your program is crucial to maintaining a healthy body weight and preventing age-related muscle loss. Weightlifting and other bodyweight exercises are examples of strength training that can greatly increase muscle size and function as well as muscle strength. Strength training can also aid in weight loss by increasing your metabolism and decreasing body fat, both of which can raise your daily caloric expenditure.

2. Unite

It can be difficult to start an exercise or good eating regimen on your own. Getting in a partner with a friend, coworker, or relative may increase your likelihood of following through on your strategy and reaching your wellness objectives. For instance, studies reveal that people who participate in weight-loss programs alongside friends have a much higher chance of keeping the weight off in the long run. Furthermore, exercising with friends can increase your dedication to a fitness program and increase your enjoyment of it.

3. Move more and sit less

Losing excess body fat requires burning more calories than you consume. For this reason, increasing your daily physical activity is crucial when attempting to reduce weight. For instance, spending a lot of time sitting at your work may hinder your attempts to lose weight. You can combat this by simply getting up from your desk and going for a five-minute stroll once each hour at work to increase your level of activity. According to research, wearing a Fitbit or pedometer to count your steps can help you lose weight by raising your caloric expenditure and level of exercise.

Establish a reasonable step goal for yourself using a pedometer or Fitbit depending on your present level of exercise. After that, progressively increase your daily step total to 7,000–10,000 or higher, depending on your general health.

4. Increase your protein consumption

Consuming adequate high-quality protein in your diet is essential for halting or reversing age-related muscle loss in addition to helping you lose weight. After the age of 20, your resting metabolic rate (RMR), or the number of calories you burn while at rest, drops by 1% to 2% every ten years. This is linked to the loss of muscle with aging.

A diet high in protein, however, can help stop or even reverse muscle loss. Increasing your dietary protein intake can aid in weight loss and help you maintain it off over time, according to numerous studies. Furthermore, studies indicate that older persons require more protein than younger adults do, which emphasizes the significance of including foods high in protein in your meals and snacks.

5. Consult a nutritionist

It can be challenging to find an eating schedule that nourishes your body and aids in weight loss. You can find the most effective strategy to reduce excess body fat without needing to adhere to an unduly restrictive diet by speaking with a qualified dietitian. A dietician can also help and mentor you during your weight loss process.

Working with a dietician can help you lose weight more successfully and sustain it over time, according to research. The outcomes can be much better than trying to reduce weight on your own.

6. Increase home cooking

Those who cook and eat more of their meals at home typically maintain a healthier diet and weigh less than those who don't, according to numerous studies. You have complete control over what ingredients go into and are left out of your recipes when you cook at home. It also allows you to try out new, healthful foods that catch your attention.

If you go out to dine for most of your meals, cook one or two meals a week at home to begin with, and then progressively increase the number until you're cooking more at home than you are.

7. Consume more veggies

Fruits and vegetables are abundant in nutrients that are essential to your health, and including them in your diet is an easy, scientifically proven method of losing extra weight. For instance, an analysis of ten research revealed that a 0.14-inch (0.36-cm) decrease in women's waist circumference was linked to every daily serving increase of vegetables. In a different study, 26,340 men and women between the ages of 35 and 65 were found to have lower body fat, waist circumferences, and body weights who ate fruits and vegetables.

8. Get a personal coach

Those who are new to exercising might particularly benefit from working with a personal trainer, since they will teach you the proper form to encourage weight reduction and prevent injuries. Personal trainers can also encourage you to exercise more by holding you responsible. They might even help you feel better about working out. One-on-one personal training for one hour each week boosted motivation to exercise and raised levels of physical activity, according to a 10-week study involving 129 adults.

9. Reduce your reliance on quick food

Consuming convenience foods on a regular basis, such as candy, fast food, and processed snacks, is linked to weight gain and may make it more difficult to lose weight. Foods that are considered convenient often have a high calorie content and a low content of vital nutrients such as fiber, protein, vitamins, and minerals. For this reason, processed foods like fast food are frequently referred to as "empty calories." Reducing your intake of convenience foods and substituting them with nutrient-dense whole foods for wholesome meals and snacks is a wise strategy for weight loss.

10. Discover a hobby or pastime you enjoy.

It might be challenging to stick to a long-term fitness regimen. It's crucial to partake in things you enjoy because of this. For instance, if you enjoy being with people, consider joining a jogging club or group sport like soccer to get regular exercise. If you're more of a lone wolf, consider swimming, biking, walking, or hiking.

11. Consult a medical professional

It may be necessary to rule out medical disorders like hypothyroidism and polycystic ovary syndrome (PCOS) if you are not losing weight while being physically active and eating a nutritious diet. This could be particularly relevant if you have relatives who suffer from these ailments. Inform your healthcare professional about your symptoms so they can choose the appropriate course of testing to rule out any underlying medical disorders that may be causing your weight loss difficulties.

12. Adopt a diet heavy in whole foods

Eating a diet high in whole foods is one of the easiest methods to make sure that your body gets the nutrients it needs to thrive. Whole foods are rich in nutrients that are necessary for sustaining a healthy body weight, such as fiber, protein, and healthy fats. These include vegetables, fruits, nuts, seeds, chicken, fish, legumes, and grains. Whole-food-based diets, both plant-based and animal-based diets, have been linked to weight loss in numerous studies.

13. Consume less at night.

Eating less calories at night has been linked to both maintaining a healthy weight and losing excess body fat, according to numerous research. Over a 6-year period, individuals who consumed more calories at supper had a more than two-fold increased risk of obesity compared to those who consumed more calories earlier in the day, according to a study including 1,245 participants. A person's risk of developing metabolic syndrome, a collection of ailments that includes elevated blood sugar and increased abdominal fat, was also considerably higher for those who consumed more calories during supper. Your risk of heart disease, diabetes, and stroke is increased if you have metabolic syndrome.

Consuming most of your calories at breakfast and lunch and keeping your dinner lighter could be a beneficial strategy to help you lose weight.

14. Pay attention to your body type

While body weight is a useful measure of health, it's also crucial to consider your body composition, or the proportions of fat and fat-free mass in your body. Muscle mass is a crucial indicator of general health, particularly in the elderly. Your objective should be to reduce excess fat and gain more muscle. You can calculate your body fat percentage in a variety of methods. To find out if you're gaining muscle and losing fat, you can measure your thighs, chest, biceps, calves, and waist.

15. Use healthy hydration methods

Beverages that are high in calories and added sugars include soda, juices, sports drinks, sweetened coffee beverages, and pre-made smoothies. Consuming beverages with added sugar, particularly those made with high-fructose corn syrup, has been directly associated with weight gain as well as diseases like diabetes, heart disease, obesity, and fatty liver disease. Drinking water and herbal tea instead of sugary drinks will help you lose weight and lower your chance of getting the chronic illnesses listed above.

16. Select the appropriate supplements

Taking the appropriate vitamins may assist provide you with the energy you need to accomplish your goals if you're feeling worn out and unmotivated. Your body's capacity to absorb specific nutrients decreases with age, which raises the possibility of shortages. For instance, studies reveal that individuals over 50 frequently have folate and vitamin B12 deficiencies, two elements required for the synthesis of energy. B vitamin deficiencies, such as B12 deficiency, can impair mood, lead to fatigue, and impede weight reduction. Because of this, taking a high-quality B-complex vitamin can help lower the risk of insufficiency in people over 50.

17. Minimize sugar additions

For weight loss at any age, limiting foods high in added sugar is essential. These items include sweetened beverages, sweets, cakes, cookies, ice cream, sweetened yogurts, and sugary cereals. The simplest approach to find out if a food item has added sugar is to check the ingredient labels because sugar is added to a wide variety of foods, including things like bread, salad dressing, and tomato sauce that you might not think of. Check the nutrition information label for "added sugars" or look for common sweeteners like agave, high-fructose corn syrup, and cane sugar in the ingredient list.

18. Boost the quality of your sleep

Your attempts to lose weight may suffer if you don't get enough good sleep. Numerous studies have demonstrated that insufficient sleep raises the risk of obesity and may make it more difficult to lose weight. For instance, a 2-year study involving 245 women showed that those who slept seven hours or more every night had a 33 percent greater chance of losing weight compared to those who slept fewer than seven hours. Success in losing weight was also linked to higher-quality sleep. Reduce the amount of light in your bedroom, avoid using your phone or watching TV just before bed, and try to obtain the recommended 7 to 9 hours of sleep each night.

19. Give intermittent fasting a try.

An eating pattern known as intermittent fasting involves just eating for a predetermined amount of time each day. The 16/8 approach, which involves eating within an 8-hour window and then fasting for 16 hours, is the most often used kind of intermittent fasting. Several studies have demonstrated that weight loss is facilitated by intermittent fasting. Furthermore, a few studies on animals and test tubes indicate that intermittent fasting may help the elderly by extending life, delaying the aging process, and halting alterations to the mitochondria, the sections of your cells that produce energy.

20. Take greater care

Practicing mindful eating can help you lose weight and foster a better connection with food. Eating mindfully entails being more aware of your food and eating habits. It helps you gain a greater knowledge of how food affects your mood and overall wellbeing, as well as your hunger and fullness cues. Numerous researches have shown that adopting mindful eating practices enhances eating habits and encourages weight loss. While there are no set guidelines for mindful eating, some easy ways to incorporate it into your life include eating slowly, focusing on the flavor and aroma of each bite, and recording your feelings as you eat.

7.14: Expert View Fourteen:

Another panel of experts have come up with 20 realistic approaches to crack the weight loss secret. So, giving attention to them should be a judicious decision.

1.   **Get moving more**

The fundamental idea behind weight loss is to burn more calories than you take in. Sedentary lifestyles have been connected in some study to a higher risk of obesity, cardiovascular disease, and overall worse health. A major contributing element to the sedentary lifestyles of many individuals is working in a profession that requires a lot of sitting, such as being an office worker, driver, or cashier. Nonetheless, research indicates that people may decrease the amount of time they spend sitting and maybe improve their general health by taking little breaks every 30 minutes.

2.   **Important to ensure high-quality sleep.**

Several studies have shown a link between obesity and inadequate or poor-quality sleep. More specifically, studies point to a link between an elevated risk of obesity and shorter sleep duration and worse sleep quality. To reduce the risk of obesity, getting adequate good-quality sleep is essential. People may assist their general health and weight control goals by making sure they get enough sleep.

3.   **Never miss a meal**

Avoiding meal skipping may be more beneficial for weight loss than initially perceived. While it might appear advantageous in terms of reducing calorie intake, skipping meals can actually hinder weight loss efforts. Studies suggest that there may be a connection between obesity and missing breakfast, meaning that this behavior may actually lead to weight growth rather than decrease.

4.   **Take advantage of the commute**

If you want to increase your daily physical activity without putting in a lot of effort, think about making little changes to your commute. You may promote more mobility and exercise by, for example, parking your car further away from your place of employment or getting off public transit one stop early than normal. These extra calories burnt from these kinds of exercises will help you keep your weight in check.

5.   Enjoy activity

Finding an activity that you love doing is essential for long-term sustained involvement, according to several research. Finding enjoyment in exercise, whether it be via weightlifting, yoga, or tennis, helps keep people motivated and see it as a recreational activity rather than a work or duty.

6.   Involve a friend

It can be beneficial to involve a friend who has similar goals. It may be advantageous to include a buddy with like objectives. Studies show that adding a social component to weight reduction initiatives can improve plan adherence and foster better weight maintenance than going it alone.

7.   Alter the snacks you eat.

When you're hungry, think about reaching for healthy options like nuts rather than sweet confections. Studies show that eating reasonable amounts of nuts daily has no discernible effect on body weight, whereas sugary snacks are more likely to cause weight gain.

8.   Identify attainable goals

People should refrain from trying to lose weight quickly or putting too much pressure on themselves to meet unrealistic exercise goals. High expectations can breed disappointment, which may lead to a lack of commitment to diet and exercise regimens if results are not seen right away. It is preferable for people to make incremental advancements toward their ultimate goals by establishing smaller, more manageable milestones along the way.

9.   Engage in resistance training

There is evidence from several studies that people lose muscular mass and strength as they age. As such, adding weightlifting and strength training to an older adult's exercise plan can help them maintain a healthy body weight. Moreover, resistance training contributes to improved bone strength, reducing the risk of injuries and facilitating adherence to the exercise routine.

10.   Include exercise equipment

People can track their daily step count using a pedometer or wristwatch, which can be encouraging when they see a steady increase in their daily step total. Furthermore, step counting helps people determine how many calories they burn each day with greater accuracy, which makes calculating their daily caloric needs for weight reduction easier.

11.   Prioritize protein intake

Studies show that older persons may benefit most from increasing their protein intake while trying to reduce weight. By incorporating higher levels of protein into their diet, individuals in this demographic may experience greater fat loss while preserving more muscle mass compared to those who consume lower amounts of protein.

12.   Manage stress levels

Studies have demonstrated a correlation between elevated stress levels and an increased tendency for food cravings and overeating. People who are under a lot of stress frequently resort to food as a consolation, which can make it difficult to lose weight. Moreover, stress triggers the release of cortisol, a hormone linked to weight gain, particularly in the abdominal and facial areas. By actively reducing stress levels, individuals can support their weight management goals and maintain a healthier body weight.

13.   Emphasize fruits and vegetables in your diet

There is evidence from observational research that a higher fruit and vegetable intake is positively correlated with better muscular function. These nutrient-rich foods not only tend to be low in calories, but they also provide a plethora of essential nutrients that support optimal bodily functions. Furthermore, incorporating fruits and vegetables into your diet may contribute to a decreased risk of various health conditions.

14.   To lose weight, go for whole grains.

When aiming to shed extra pounds, it is beneficial to prepare meals using wholesome ingredients. When it comes to your diet, choose whole grains over processed meals. Research indicates that incorporating whole grains into your meals can lead to a notable reduction in overall energy intake and body weight, particularly in overweight adults. By making this simple dietary switch, you can support your weight loss efforts and improve your overall health.

15.   Consider hiring a personal trainer

Lack of motivation can often hinder weight loss progress, especially for individuals over the age of 50. Nonetheless, hiring a personal trainer might offer the assistance and direction required to get beyond this challenge. Personal trainers offer accountability and expertise in recommending effective weight loss strategies.

16.   Take up mild workouts like yoga.

Some research suggests that adding low-impact exercise to a weight loss regimen may be beneficial. Low impact workouts like yoga, tai chi, and Pilates might be helpful for people who might not be able to engage in more physically demanding activities. These workouts support weight reduction attempts while offering a reduced intensity option. They provide a different option for people who want to lose weight but might be unable to engage in greater impact activities due to restrictions or personal preferences. People may work toward their weight reduction objectives in a way that best fits their needs and skills by adopting these mild exercise methods.

17.   Practice mindful eating

People often multitask while eating, doing tasks like working or watching television. But when the emphasis moves away from the actual act of eating, this habit may result in overindulging. When people are less attentive to their body's signals, they may continue to consume food even after feeling full. Using mindful eating practices can be a very effective way to lose weight. By being fully present and attentive while eating, individuals can better tune into their body's cues and make more conscious choices about their food intake. By promoting a better understanding of hunger and fullness, this technique eventually aids with weight control.

18.   Eliminate sugary beverages from your diet

Consuming soda and other fizzy sugary drinks, as well as ostensibly healthful choices like store-bought smoothies, can result in a high intake of added sugar. This contributes extra calories to the diet, which might hinder weight loss attempts. Studies indicate a potential link between high-sugar beverages and a number of health issues, such as diabetes, heart disease, and fatty liver disease. Opting for healthier options, such as water or herbal teas, can aid in weight reduction. These choices support a healthy calorie intake overall in addition to aiding with thirst relief.

19.   Reduce eating out

Finding out exactly what's in a dish at a restaurant might be difficult at times. Hidden ingredients, additional fats, and sugars are commonly found in restaurant dishes, which may lead to unintentional calorie consumption. People who choose to cook more often at home have more control over the ingredients and cooking techniques. This encourages improved general health and well-being by giving them the ability to make healthier decisions and have a better grasp of what they are ingesting.

20.   Undergo testing

It is advised that those over 50 who are having difficulty losing weight get advice from a healthcare professional for a comprehensive assessment. A doctor can do a number of tests to rule out the possibility of issues that are making the effort futile.

According to the expert, if someone is putting efforts for shedding the extra pounds for roughly six months having no visible outcome, they need to take professional guidance.

7.15: Expert View Fifteen:

According to the expert, if someone is putting efforts for shedding the extra pounds for roughly six months having no visible outcome, they need to take professional guidance.

Some professional advices on how to lose weight after 50.

1.   Strength training

Strength training is essential for maintaining muscle mass, especially as we age. By the age of 50, we may have lost around 10% of our muscular mass. This decrease in muscle mass not only affects our appearance but also impacts our metabolism.

Muscle is more metabolically active than fat, meaning it burns more calories even at rest. As a result, having a greater muscle-to-fat ratio allows us to burn more energy even while we're sitting or not actively moving. To build and maintain muscle mass, regular exercise is crucial.

Although there are advantages to all types of exercise, gaining muscle is especially facilitated by strength training, such as lifting weights. This is true for both men and women. A review of studies published in Sports Medicine in 2021 found that women aged 50 and older can also reap numerous benefits from strength training.

To incorporate strength training into your routine, aim for two to three weight training sessions per week. This frequency allows for adequate recovery and muscle growth. If you're new to strength training, start with lesser weights or resistance bands and gradually increase the intensity as you gain comfort and strength.

In addition to building muscle, strength training offers several other advantages, including improved bone health, increased strength and endurance, enhanced balance and stability, and a reduced risk of injury. It can also help with weight loss and overall well-being.

2.   The 200-calorie rule.

Your daily calorie requirements tend to drop slightly as you become older. Many people, however, continue to consume the same quantity of food without accounting for this shift. After the age of 50, it is suggested by the government's dietary guidelines to burn around 200 fewer daily calories.

To achieve this calorie reduction, a combination of calorie cutting and strength training is suggested. A calorie-counting program like MyFitnessPal, Cronometer, or MyNetDiary is one approach to track and limit your calorie consumption. These apps provide a convenient way to monitor your food consumption and make informed choices about your diet.

Seminal research published in the journal Obesity in 2017 engaged 249 adults aged 60 and above to assess the efficacy of diet and exercise on fat and muscle composition. Three groups of participants were formed. One group was advised to decrease 300 calories from their daily meals. Another group restricted calories while simultaneously engaging in 45 minutes of aerobic activity four times each week. The third group alternated between calorie restriction and strength training. Those who combined diet and exercise dropped the greatest weight (20 pounds on average) after 18 months. The strength-training group, on the other hand, shed more fat (18 pounds) and less muscle (just 2 pounds).

3. Drink plenty of fluids.

Staying well-hydrated by drinking plenty of fluids is not only essential for overall health but also plays a significant role in maintaining a healthy weight. Compared to adults who are well-hydrated, individuals who are dehydrated may age more quickly and have a higher chance of developing chronic illnesses.

When you drink water, your body goes through a process known as thermogenesis, in which it utilizes energy to bring the liquid to body temperature. This implies that merely drinking water can help you burn calories and enhance your metabolism. While the calorie-burning effect is little, every little amount helps to increase your overall energy expenditure.

Fluid intake is also important in the complicated process of converting carbohydrates and protein into useful energy.

When your body is properly hydrated, these metabolic processes can occur more efficiently, supporting your overall energy production and utilization.

It is typically suggested that you drink eight glasses of water every day to stay hydrated. Individual fluid requirements, on the other hand, might vary depending on factors such as activity level, environment, and personal health concerns. It's important to listen to your body's thirst signals and adjust your fluid intake accordingly.

In addition to drinking water, you can also increase your fluid intake by consuming foods with high water content, such as fruits and vegetables. These types of food not only help you stay hydrated, but they also provide important minerals, fiber, and antioxidants that promote overall health.

Keep in mind that water is the finest and most natural hydration option. While other beverages like tea, coffee, and herbal infusions can contribute to your fluid intake, it's important to be mindful of their caffeine and sugar content, as excessive consumption of these substances may have negative effects on health.

Prioritizing hydration by drinking enough water and consuming water-rich meals will help you feel better overall, aid in weight loss, and contribute to optimal biological functions.

4.   Cardio and HIIT Exercise

Maintaining a healthy weight and supporting general well-being requires a combination of strength-building exercises and cardiac activity. While strength training helps maintain muscle mass and increases metabolism, cardiovascular training has its own set of advantages.

According to experts like William Yancy Jr., a combination of strength-building activities and cardio exercise is recommended. Strength training aids in the preservation and growth of muscle, which is necessary for maintaining a higher metabolic rate. Muscles are metabolically active structures that, even at rest, burn more calories than fat. Strength-building activities, such as lifting weights or utilizing resistance bands, can assist improve muscle mass while also supporting a healthy metabolism.

However, cardio exercise shouldn't be overlooked. Cardiovascular activities, such as brisk walking, running, swimming, or cycling, provide significant health advantages. They help improve cardiovascular fitness, strengthen the heart and lungs, enhance circulation, and promote endurance. Cardio activity also helps with calorie burning and weight loss.

Adults should get at least 150 minutes of moderate-intensity cardiac activity every week, according to the Centers for Disease Control and Prevention (CDC). This may be accomplished by exercises such as brisk walking, in which you maintain a moderate speed while raising your heart rate and breathing rate. Alternatively, you can engage in higher-intensity, shorter-duration exercises such as jogging or high-intensity interval training (HIIT).

You may attain a well-rounded workout regimen that promotes muscle preservation, stimulates metabolism, improves cardiovascular health, and aids in weight control by mixing strength-building exercises and aerobic activity. Remember to listen to your body, begin slowly, and gradually increase the intensity and duration of your workouts as you develop.

5.   Reduce Your Sugar Intake

Reducing your consumption of sweets and added sugars is definitely a critical feature of keeping a healthy weight, and there are specific reasons why it's important, particularly as you age.

Reduce your intake of sweets and added sugars to help avoid excessive insulin spikes and the development of insulin resistance. This, in turn, can help with weight control and make reaching weight reduction objectives simpler.

It's crucial to understand that cutting back on sweets is about more than just lowering your calorie consumption. It also talks about how sugar affects hormonal changes, insulin levels, and the danger of developing insulin resistance. You may promote general health, maintain a healthy weight, and minimize the risk of related issues by making better choices and choosing meals low in added sugars.

6.   To Cut Down on Late-Night Munching

To cut down on late-night munching and encourage healthy habits:

·   Establish consistent meal times: Maintain a consistent eating pattern throughout the day, including scheduled meals and snacks. This can help regulate hunger and prevent excessive cravings later in the evening.

·   Practice mindful eating: When you do eat, pay attention to your food selections and quantities. Pay attention to your body's hunger and fullness cues, and strive for well-balanced meals rich in protein, fiber, healthy fats, and carbs.

·   Create a calming bedtime routine: calming activities before bed, including as reading, having a bath, or practicing meditation, can help reduce stress and lessen the need for late-night snacking caused by emotional or boredom eating.

·   Choose healthier alternatives: If you find yourself needing a late-night snack, go for something healthy like a piece of fruit, a handful of nuts, or a cup of herbal tea. These options are fewer in calories and give some fullness without interfering with sleep or generating excessive calorie consumption.

You may promote your overall well-being, maintain a healthier body weight, and lower the risk of negative health outcomes associated with late-night snacking by avoiding late-night munching and creating better behaviors.

7.   Know your Medication

If you are having difficulty losing weight while taking any drugs, get medical assistance to explore your particular weight management alternatives. Your doctor may be able to recommend alternate drugs that do not cause weight gain.

It's crucial to remember that everyone's reaction to drugs differs, so it's critical to check with a healthcare expert who can give tailored recommendations based on your individual circumstances.

8.   Adequate sleep is crucial

Maintaining a regular sleep schedule is critical for weight management. Going to bed and waking up at the same time every day promotes your body's internal clock and can improve your metabolism. Sleep pattern inconsistency, with considerable fluctuations in sleep time, might affect metabolic function and potentially lead to weight gain.

 If you struggle to keep a consistent sleep routine, establishing a nighttime ritual might help. A nighttime routine alerts your body and mind that it is time to unwind and prepare for sleep. Turning off electronic devices at least an hour before bed, changing into appropriate sleepwear, practicing relaxation techniques such as deep breathing or meditation, and brushing your teeth are all examples of activities that fall into this category.

You may help your weight loss objectives by emphasizing excellent sleep hygiene and developing a consistent sleep regimen. To improve your general health, well-being, and weight-loss attempts, aim for 7-9 hours of excellent sleep every night.

9.   Watch out for your weight

Regular weight monitoring can be an effective technique for both weight reduction and weight management. Whether you choose to weigh yourself every morning or every week is a personal preference, but consistency is key. It's important to step on the scale at the same time of day for each weigh-in to get a more accurate understanding of your progress.

Two-year research found that regular weigh-ins and charting the findings can be useful for both reducing and keeping weight off. By routinely checking your weight, you can hold yourself responsible to your objectives and make necessary lifestyle changes.

Keeping track of your weight on a chart helps you to see your improvement over time. It gives you a clear picture of how well your weight reduction efforts are working and assists you in identifying any patterns or trends. This may be motivational and give useful information about which tactics are working for you.

When tracking your weight, it's important to remember that weight fluctuates naturally due to various factors like water retention, digestion, and muscle gain. Focus on the overall trend rather than day-to-day fluctuations. If you see consistent improvement over time, it means your weight loss efforts are working.

In addition to tracking your weight, it's also helpful to monitor other aspects of your health and well-being, such as body measurements, energy levels, and how your clothes fit.

These can provide you a more complete picture of your development and general health.

Remember that weight is just one aspect of health, and it's important to prioritize overall well-being and body positivity. Celebrate all of the great improvements you're making, regardless of the scale numbers.

10.   Effective Weight Loss Objectives

According to studies, effective weight loss objectives include the following critical elements:

·   Rather than a general goal of eating more fruits and vegetables, make it particular by striving to consume five servings of fruit and vegetables every day.

·   Set a concrete goal, such as tracking 10,000 steps each day on your activity tracker, to measure your progress. This way, you have a clear goal to strive toward and can track your daily progress.

·   It is critical to develop realistic and reachable objectives. Rather of committing to going to the gym every day, choose a more manageable target of three days per week. This helps you to gradually increase your fitness program without becoming overwhelmed.

·   Make sure your objectives are realistic in relation to your lifestyle and tastes. For example, if you want to cut back on soda, make a realistic target of drinking sparkling water four out of every five times. This way, you may maintain some freedom while making healthy choices.

·   Setting a definite start date for your new eating plan and noting it on your calendar gives your goal a time-bound component. This creates a sense of urgency and dedication, which makes staying on track simpler.

By adding these factors into your weight reduction objectives, you boost your chances of success and establish a clear path to your desired results.

11.   Avoid ultra-processed foods.

In a small study, participants were divided into two groups and placed on different diets to examine the effects of unprocessed foods versus ultra-processed foods on weight loss efforts. The diets were either unprocessed meals like fruits and vegetables, lean meats, and whole grains, or ultra-processed foods like cured meats, baked goods, and snack aisle items.

Participants in both groups received the same total number of calories, protein, and carbs. They were also allowed to eat as much as they wanted throughout the study period. After fourteen days, the participants switched to the opposite diet plan.

The results of the study revealed that when participants consumed ultra-processed foods, they consumed an average of 500 calories more per day compared to when they were on the unprocessed foods diet. This calorie increase resulted in weight gain rather than weight loss, emphasizing the possible harmful influence of ultra-processed meals on overall energy balance and weight control.

It is worth noting that this study was carried out in a relatively short period of time and with a small sample size. It does, however, give useful information on the possible impact of ultra-processed meals on weight loss efforts.

To support weight loss goals, it is advisable to prioritize whole, unprocessed foods and limit the consumption of ultra-processed options. This can help regulate calorie consumption, offer important nutrients, and contribute to a healthier and more lasting weight-management strategy.

12.   Motivated to exercise: avoid making excuses

Here are some tips to help you stay motivated to exercise:

·   Avoid making excuses.

·   Choose a gym near to your home for convenience.

·   Enlist the help of a workout companion to inspire and support one another.

·   Consider hiring a personal trainer for accountability and instruction.

·   Make your exercises become non-negotiable appointments.

·   Use any or all of these methods to maintain accountability and commitment to your fitness objectives on days when you're lacking motivation.

By applying these tactics, you may eliminate excuses and make regular exercise a priority in your life.

13.   Meal planning

Meal planning ahead of time is an easy approach to stick to your diet. You can prepare the required components for the following week by devoting a few hours over the weekend. Here are some pointers for efficient meal preparation:

·   Cook healthful grains ahead of time, such as quinoa or brown rice, and keep them in the fridge for rapid warming.

·   Prepare beans or lentils as a protein source or to add to salads and soups throughout the week.

·   Roast a variety of veggies that may be readily incorporated into meals or served as side dishes.

·   Grill chicken breasts or any protein of choice that can be portioned and used for numerous meals.

When you are busy during the week, having prepared items on hand saves time and promotes healthier choices.

14. Add Whole Grains into Your Diet

Including whole grains in your diet may provide extra benefits. Whole grains include the entire kernel, including the fiber-rich bran and nutrient-dense germ. This means your body will use more energy digesting them, resulting in a bigger calorie burn. In a study of 40 to 65-year-olds, changing refined white flour and rice for whole grains resulted in an increase of roughly 100 more calories expended per day, even when overall calorie consumption remained same.

You may boost your metabolism and perhaps help your weight reduction or maintenance objectives by incorporating whole grains in your meals.

15. Increase Protein Intake

Consider the following suggestions to ensure you obtain enough protein and maintain muscular health:

·   Include the following high-quality protein sources in your diet: Include foods like eggs, lean meats (like chicken, turkey, and lean cuts of cattle), fish, dairy products (like Greek yogurt and cottage cheese), legumes (like beans and lentils), and tofu or other plant-based protein sources in your diet. These meals include necessary amino acids that are required for muscle maintenance and development.

·   Consider high-quality nutritional supplements: If necessary, protein powders or protein bars can be used to boost your protein consumption. Look for goods with high-quality components and a well-balanced spectrum of necessary amino acids.

·   According to research, a greater protein diet is connected with reduced muscle mass loss over time, particularly in certain groups. Research published in The American Journal of Clinical Nutrition discovered that a higher protein diet resulted in reduced muscle mass loss in women aged 70 to 79, particularly Black women, over three years. As a result, monitor your protein consumption, especially as you become older.

·   Distribute protein intake throughout the day: Aim to include protein-rich foods in all your meals and snacks. According to research, eating similar quantities of protein at each meal can improve muscular strength and metabolism, especially in those over the age of 67.

Remember to seek the advice of a healthcare expert or qualified dietitian for individualized suggestions based on your unique needs and health objectives. They can advise you on the best protein consumption for you and help you build a well-balanced diet.

16. Be More Active

You may be surprised to learn that you do not need to engage in difficult activities alone to burn calories. The effect of walking pace on weight reduction in previously sedentary postmenopausal women was investigated in a study published in the journal Nutrients. Although overall body fat reduction happens at all walking rates, slow walkers (defined as less than 3.5 miles per hour) who are overweight saw bigger early decreases in body fat. This implies that even moderate-paced walking can help with weight loss.

Wearing an accelerometer can assist in measuring your steps and analyzing the intensity of your daily activities if you're unclear about your level of physical activity throughout the day. This gadget monitors movement and can offer information about your general level of physical activity.

17. Hara Hachi Bu

When it comes to eating, it's crucial to prioritize feeling content over eating until you're entirely stuffed. In Japanese culture, the notion of "hara hachibu" encourages eating until you are around 80% satisfied. This approach allows for mindful eating and can help prevent overeating.

The idea is to pay attention to your body's hunger and satiety signals. Pay attention to your feelings throughout meals and stop eating when you begin to feel satisfied. This gives your body time to realize that it has absorbed adequate nutrition.

By practicing mindful eating and stopping at the point of satisfaction, you can avoid the discomfort of feeling overly full and promote healthier eating habits. It's crucial to remember that this may take some time because it entails learning to recognize your body's signals and distinguish between hunger and fullness.

18. Strategies for healthy metabolism

It is critical to adapt our food and activity habits as we age to combat the potential decline in metabolism and prevent weight gain. To keep a healthy metabolism, follow the strategies such as Stay active, eat a balanced diet, stay hydrated, get enough protein, manage stress.

By adopting these lifestyle habits, you can help maintain a healthy metabolism and support your weight management goals as you age. Keep in mind that little adjustments over time may have a big influence on your overall health and well-being.

19. Avoid ALCOHOL

Consider the following advice to reduce your alcohol intake while keeping your weight-management objectives in mind:

Drink in moderation:

Moderation is key. Drink no more than one drink per day for ladies and two drinks per day for males, according to established standards.

Choose lower calorie options:

Low-calorie alcoholic beverages, such as light beers, dry wines, or spirits blended with calorie-free mixers like soda water or Diet Coke, are preferable. Sugary mixers and cocktails should be avoided since they can drastically increase calorie consumption.

Alternate with water:

To keep hydrated and limit total alcohol intake, alternate alcoholic beverages with water. This can also help you regulate your appetite and avoid overeating.

Be mindful of portion sizes:

Pay attention to portion amounts and strive to keep to normal serving quantities. Oversized glasses and heavy-handed pours should be avoided since they might lead to unintended overconsumption.

Consider non-alcoholic alternatives:

If you're concerned about the influence of alcohol on your weight-loss objectives, think about mocktails or alcohol-free beverages. These can offer a comparable social experience without the extra calories.

Remember that alcohol has different impacts on different people, so listen to your body and make decisions that match your own health objectives. If you have particular concerns or issues, you should always seek the advice of a healthcare practitioner or qualified dietitian.

7.16: Expert View Sixteen:
Ingestion of the body and spirit

Adhering to intuitive eating entails disregarding diet mentality and instead focusing on our innate signals of appetite and satiety. How could you potentially benefit?

Destroyed by an extended period of dieting? It appears that you have attempted everything to lose weight, including low-calorie, low-sugar, low-fat, low-carb, and frankly, low-satisfaction programs that have only served to exhaust you further.

If the description aligns with your interests, you might be inclined towards an entirely different approach. Decades-old intuitive eating is intended to assist individuals mired in the cycle of dieting in developing a more positive relationship with food. The concept that our bodies possess an innate understanding of what, when, and in what quantity to consume in order to maintain nourishment is fundamental. However, a lifetime of constant communication—from directives to "clean your plate" to demonstrations of super-thin models—has prevented many of us from heeding that inner voice.

The rejection of the rules and restrictions inherent in a diet paradigm by intuitive eating frequently results in a cyclical pattern of weight gain and loss. Approximately 80% of individuals who lose a substantial quantity of weight will likely regain some or all of it within a year, according to the available evidence. Conversely, intuitive eating promotes the practice of eating only when one feels hungry and ceasing when one is replete. Additionally, satisfaction derived from consuming one's food is considered, which paradoxically could result in weight loss.

"Continually gaining and losing weight for years and years is a difficult way to live and can be counterproductive," says Emily Blake, a dietitian at Brigham and Women's Hospital, which is affiliated with Harvard. "Intuitive eating is a framework that integrates mind and body and encourages you to trust in your own ability to feed yourself."

A balanced strategy

A second fundamental tenet of intuitive eating is the rejection of the notion that foods are "good" or "bad" by nature. Pizza, pasta, and burgers have been removed from the evil list. Similarly, fruits and salads do not constitute "better."

"What people find over time is they end up craving a balance of foods," Blake asserts. "Your self-confidence will increase significantly as you gain the ability to consume foods that comfort you physically, devoid of any emotional distress or guilt." After detaching the moral dimension of food, one begins to discern that although occasional cravings for less-than-nutritious options do occur, fruits and vegetables are frequently desired as well.

Conversely, certain individuals erroneously perceive intuitive eating as an unrestricted food allowance, according to Nancy Oliveira, superintendent of the Nutrition and Wellness Service at Brigham and Women's Hospital and a registered dietitian.

"When people have food freedom, some may choose more ultra-processed, 'craveable' foods," according to Oliveira. "It is somewhat difficult. It does improve your overall relationship with food, but it must be complemented by sound nutritional knowledge and common sense. You must understand that consuming potato chips throughout the day will not improve your mood in the long term.

Feisty versus replete

Many individuals who are attempting to embrace intuitive eating face a significant obstacle in reacquainting themselves with the bodily signals that indicate appetite or satiety and reacting appropriately. "Most people recognize hunger pangs, but a lot of people struggle with fullness," according to Blake. "It's not really the American way to recognize being full."

Perhaps it is immediately apparent that your dizziness or stomach rumbling indicate the urgent need for sustenance. However, feeling filled is not the same as knowing you've overindulged and are now gasping for air.

"Occasionally, the phrase 'comfortably un-hungry' is employed," Oliveira explains. "You feel mentally satisfied because you chose exactly what you wanted to eat, and you feel better afterward, with more energy."

Blake suggests establishing a check-in point throughout your meal—for instance, at the midpoint—and pausing momentarily to evaluate your appetite and level of fullness. If you feel as though you may be filled, refrigerate your plate. "If you're still hungry 20 minutes later, you can have more—it's not a big deal," according to her. "This facilitates your development of comfort with those cues." "Developing a skill is similar to gaining muscle; however, the process will require a considerable amount of time."

Mind-body advantages

Weight loss may be the result of intuitive eating, particularly if heeding hunger and satiety signals motivates one to consume fewer calories. A 2019 review of research published in the journal Obesity Reviews analyzed the dietary patterns of nearly 1,500 individuals across ten studies. Individuals who adhered to an intuitive eating plan experienced comparable weight loss to those who followed conventional weight-loss diets, and greater weight loss than those who did not alter their eating patterns.

However, Blake and Oliveira stress that intuitive feeding does not aim to promote weight loss. Instead, it may be more practical to develop the ability to recognize and adhere to your body's "set point," which is the point at which your weight drops naturally while you provide it with sufficient nutrition and allow for some flexibility in terms of exercise and diet. According to a study published in the International Journal of nutrition Disorders in 2021, intuitive nutrition is associated with improved body image and self-esteem.

"If people have a tough relationship with food stemming from a long history of dieting, they can feel better emotionally," according to Blake. "This also makes it easier to accept where their body is in terms of weight."

Strategies for Achieving Success

Are you intrigued? Oliveira and Blake provide the following suggestions for living an intuitive diet.

Practice mindfulness while eating. This is accomplished through the use of slow chewing, pauses between bites, and the avoidance of displays and other electronic devices.

Reduce your sense of remorse. "I don't care if you eat pepperoni pizza for every meal for an entire week," Blake asserts. "Don't beat yourself up for any of your choices."

Maintain a food journal without performing calorie counting. Monitor how you feel, when you feel hungry and full, what you consume, and when you feel satisfied. "You're shifting focus from nutrient and calorie content to why and what you're eating, and that's useful self-reflection," Oliveira asserts.

Examine your emotions. Consider whether the urge to eat promptly after your last meal is motivated by boredom, stress, or genuine hunger. This may be the result of consuming emotionally. "Maybe you need a nice cup of tea, a warm bath, or a walk instead," Oliveira advises.

Avoid fixating on weight loss. "If you're focused on the scale, you're not going to listen to your body," Oliveira asserts. "At least for a month, just focus on your body's signals."

Maintain electricity. For instance, missing a meal throughout the day and returning home to an unopened carton of cookies increases the likelihood of binge eating. "Part of intuitive eating is making sure you're eating enough over all so you're not trying to practice these principles while starving," Blake asserts.

Attempt to obtain support. For further guidance, consult a registered dietitian or health coach.

Exercise patience. Regaining the ability to rely on your body's signals requires time. "There's going to be a lot of trial and error where you feel intuitive eating isn't working," Oliveira asserts.

Four misconceptions about nutrition that can derail a healthy diet

Despite the recent proliferation of nutrition information supported by scientific evidence, certain dietary fallacies continue to persist. However, these misunderstandings may prevent us from consuming essential nutrients, derailment of a healthy diet, according to Nancy Oliveira, a dietitian at Brigham and Women's Hospital.

She claims that social media is primarily to blame. Prior to the proliferation of nutritional "advice" on social media platforms such as Facebook and YouTube, individuals relied more heavily on reputable health information sources and government guidelines. "All of a sudden, these voices are advising against consuming particular foods." "People are completely perplexed," Oliveira explains. "It misleads and distracts them from what really matters."

Oliveira explains which beliefs appear to be the most widespread and why they are false:

Myth: Dairy milk is unhealthier than plant-based milk.

Alternative milks such as soy, oat, almond, and others are highly suitable for individuals who have lactose intolerance or an aversion to cow's milk. A cup of the latter, however, contains approximately 10 grams of protein and 25 percent of the daily calcium requirement, whereas plant milks typically contain considerably less protein. Oliveira advises consumers to scrutinize product labels, as all milk varieties may contain protein, calcium, and vitamin D fortifications. "If those nutrients are important to you, be sure to double-check, as amounts can vary among brands," according to her.

Myth: Completely avoid carbohydrates.

 Although carbohydrates are vital to a healthy diet, the type of carbohydrates consumed is significant. Reduce your intake of refined carbohydrates, including those found in white breads, cakes, pastries, and chips, as they cause blood sugar spikes. Complex carbohydrates, which are found in fruits, vegetables, whole cereals, and legumes, provide sustained energy and prolong satiety. "Good carbohydrates exist, and our bodies require them," Oliveira explains.

Myth: Frozen fruits and vegetables are less nutritious than fresh ones.

Enzyme loss commences as soon as the produce is harvested. However, freezer-safe varieties are commonly flash-frozen, which effectively maintains vitamin content and hinders rapid decomposition.

Myth: Fat is unhealthy.

Even decades after the low-fat mania of the 1990s peaked, there are still those who maintain the view that all fats are forbidden. However, saturated fat, found in animal products like red meat, is a less-than-healthy option that can obstruct arteries. Incorporating unsaturated fats from sources such as avocados, nuts, seeds, olive oil, and fatty salmon into one's diet rather than saturated fats safeguards cardiovascular health by increasing concentrations of HDL (good) cholesterol while decreasing LDL (bad) cholesterol. A high fat intake, especially of saturated fat, raises cholesterol levels in the body, but cholesterol per se does not have nearly the same effect. Be wary of products bearing the label "no cholesterol"; they may contain an excessive amount of saturated fat despite being plant-based.

7.17: Expert View Seventeen:
Dealing with the problem mentally:

Every January, we wish each other a happy and healthy New Year.

We think the two go hand in hand. After all, how can you be happy if you have all the aches, pains, and illnesses that come with getting older? Actually, how you live your life has a lot to do with how happily you age.

Our feelings, like anger, love, pride, and so on, are what make us human. But if we can't control our bad feelings, they can also make us unhappy. No matter what age you are, being able to focus on good feelings is important. As you get older, it becomes even more important. Studies show that having good feelings may actually make you live longer. They make you happier and stronger. A strong social network is important for staying healthy as you age, and a cheerful outlook always brings people together.

Even though no one is ever truly happy, it is possible to direct your feelings in that way. To find more happiness now and in the years to come, try to develop these four good emotions.

1. Peace and calm

Where is the most peaceful place you can think of? A calm beach with soft breezes and a blue sea that sparkles. A calm and peaceful place. Think about how happy you'd be if your mind was calm and peaceful like that place. But if you brought all of your stuff with you to the beach, your island paradise wouldn't be as peaceful. Your mind isn't either when you've been holding on to years of hurt, anger, and sadness. This memory of the past is like a rope that will hold you down. So, accept it and learn from it. Get up and go. You should go to that beach.

2. Making peace

If you hold a grudge, you'll only feel stress, anger, and pressure to judge. Not being able to let go of mistakes, even your own, will keep you from being happy. Most likely, you've racked up a good number of them after decades of living, working, and having complicated relationships. Why be hard on yourself about the past? Learn from your mistakes and use what you've learned in the present and the future. When you forgive someone, you need to admit when you were wrong, learn from it, and move on.

3. Joy

A visit from an old friend, good news, or a thank-you note from the heart in your junk mail can make any day better. It's when something great just happens out of the blue, but you won't feel it if you don't notice the good things that happen all the time. To live a happy life, you need to know yourself. It means taking the time to enjoy the good things in your life all the time, not just sometimes. Ask yourself, "What can I do to make my life more joyful?" After that, make it happen.

4. Thank you

The best luck doesn't come from a cookie; it comes from being aware and kind. Consciously being thankful every day is helpful. So, value the kindness people show you and the time and work they put into making you happy. Say thank you. Tell them how you feel. Being thankful comes to life when you share it. You should also be kind to yourself more.

Being happy as you get older is a choice, not a coincidence, and it depends a lot on how much you value life's pleasures. You can make good things happen and enjoy every minute of it by focusing on good feelings and learning where happiness comes from.

7.18: Case Study - what does the real examples say?

After exploring the pros and cons of all the solutions to weight loss regimen, it will be the right time for us to associate your physical condition and the right kind of approach to find the holy grail of your weight loss query through some case studies.

7.18.1: Case Study - 1:

In her late 40s, in Omaha, Nebraska-based pharmaceutical sales professional and mother of two, Loralee Coulter, started to discover that she was gaining weight, according to A Mom on the Road and Jenny Craig. "I wasn't eating enough fresh stuff," admits Coulter, who was normally no heavier than 170 pounds at 5'10". "I would get a sub sandwich, but not long after that, I would get hungry again.

Or else I would go the entire day without eating and then overindulge at supper.

To make matters worse, she had trouble exercising due to a foot injury she sustained in 2016. "I had gained up to 228 pounds by the time I turned 50 in 2017," Coulter states. "After viewing the photos from our family's trip to Disney World, I felt compelled to take action. I therefore made the decision to work for Jenny Craig.

Coulter claims that a greater understanding of portion control and how much she was actually eating was what she needed from a weight loss strategy. "Oh my gosh, I was eating a lot more than I thought I was," she admits after beginning to follow their regimen. Additionally, she started documenting her food intake using an app called My Net Diary that tracked calories, allowing her to gradually wean herself off of Jenny Craig meals and create a daily eating plan. She asserts, "You can't stay on a 'diet' forever."

Coulter reached her target weight of 176 pounds by the end of 2017 and has been there ever since. For long-term health, "the key is to learn how to eat in a balanced, more nutritious way," she advises.

7.18.2: Case Study - 2 :100 Pounds Lost In spite of disability

Lynn Burgess had battled with her weight for a long time due to her rheumatoid disease. However, she became less and less active when her RA got so bad that she had to go on disability in her mid-40s. The Chicago-area resident Burgess, 60, adds, "Being at home all the time, I also ate a lot more and didn't cook healthy meals like I should." Burgess discovered in 2017 that, at barely 4'11", she weighed well over 200 pounds and needed to shed over 100 pounds. "I had to try even though it was really intimidating."

She signed back up with Weight Watchers, which had assisted her in the past with lesser weight losses. "I made the decision that I wouldn't give up even if I occasionally won or didn't lose because that's inevitable," the woman explains. "I don't think it's the plan you use so much as the commitment to follow it," the person who used Weight Watchers said. Burgess lost 100 pounds over the course of roughly a year and a half, and she has maintained her weight loss for the last two years. "I felt amazing once I started noticing the difference in my clothes and when I looked in the mirror after gaining about 20 or 30 pounds," she says. "It enabled me to persevere."

7.18.3: Case Study - 3: Giving Up on Dad

Mr. Todd Bentsen is a father of two and a communications professional located in Washington, DC. He used to not really struggle with his weight. He stands just under six feet tall and has carried a weight of about 175 pounds for the majority of his adult life. Next was COVID. Bentsen, who is now sixty, frequently felt at home. "I was drinking whatever was in front of me and eating whatever my teenage kid was eating. I was almost 200 pounds in three months," he claims. "I could no longer fit into my clothes." Furthermore, the fact that your metabolism decreases with age is not a joke.

He registered for the Noom app-based weight loss program in July 2020. While Bentsen acknowledged and adhered to Noom's behavior-focused instructions, he claims that monitoring his eating patterns was the most beneficial aspect of the program. They determine how many calories you are allowed to consume each day based on your weight loss objectives. 1,400 was mine," he states. Before long, he realized just how much he had been absorbing without even noticing. He responds, "I don't know that I realized how much," while knowing that some foods are high in calories. "Although baguettes are ridiculously high in calories, I adore baguette sandwiches from the neighborhood French bakery. I've become more mindful and deliberate in my diet.

December 2020 saw him attain his target weight of 177. "I wanted an approach I could stick with, but I probably could have hit it much faster had I been stricter with myself," he adds. Using a Doctor for Weight Loss Jamie Cohen, a business entrepreneur in Connecticut, was in her late 40s and in excellent condition. Mother of two high school students adds, "I had done an elimination diet where I figured out a bunch of foods, I had sensitivities to." "I performed well if I avoided certain foods. I was feeling fantastic, sleeping soundly, and had lost weight.

Subsequently, Cohen had multiple stressors simultaneously, coinciding with her 50th birthday: family health issues, academic challenges for one of her children, and the onset of menopause. She soon discovered that she had quietly gained 225 pounds. The 5'6" Cohen claims, "I was experiencing every single menopause symptom, in addition to a lot of intestinal issues." "I saw a gastroenterologist, and he recommended that I join a medical weight loss program."

The physician overseeing the program prescribed a daily or weekly calorie intake based on Cohen's weight and amount of activity. "I quickly realized I was letting a lot more refined carbs and sugar sneak back into my diet, even though I thought I wasn't eating that much," she adds. It was a number of small changes, such as adding extra sugar and milk to my tea. Then, as I put on weight, I would feel self-conscious when I looked in the mirror, drink more tea that was very sweetened and milky, and feel horrible about myself.

Cohen started tracking her food intake and activity using the Lose It! app. I'm noticing that I'm giving up munching. When I'm hungry, I eat. I'm paying attention to my body's cues," she declares. With the assistance of online barre and Pilates sessions, she has so far dropped 47 pounds and at least three sizes. "I'm working on turning everything into muscle, so even though I still weigh more than I would like to, my shape is so much different and I'm stronger," she adds.

7.19: Advice from a Physician

 How can you achieve the same outcomes as these people? Expert Srinath offers some advice. "Calorie in, calorie out is the key to weight loss," she states. "You need to generate a daily 500-calorie deficit, which is difficult to do with food or activity alone, in order to lose one pound every week. You require both. Keep an eye on your meals. All our weight loss success stories have one thing in common: they were simply unaware of how much they were consuming. "To get started, I suggest using an app like Lose It! or MyFitnessPal to track your food intake," adds Srinath.

Conclusion

After making a labyrinthine journey of different routes, we have come to the culmination phase about our detailed discussion. In short, we have initiated our expedition with food. In fact, we dissected the food domain in considerable detail, encompassing all the components and types that would atomically pile up the building blocks of the food pyramid. The objective was to give the reader a grasp over the whole landscape so the enlightened reader can discern among the food elements that would provide them their individual nutritional support. We also delved into the reality check for women's weight issue. We compared the male and female weight gain complexity and found that women are at a bit of disadvantage with shedding the weight. Apart from that, we also raised the question and found that graceful aging is not totally a myth; with perseverance, one can turn it into a reality. Meanwhile, it was also observed that aging has its own charm - one can detach themselves from the unnecessary complication of life. Then we got our hands dirty by prodding into the weight gain hypotheses. It was observed that hormone plays the pivotal role in determining the aging as well as the weight aspects. Unfortunately, it is a regretful context for women to reach the age mark of 50 with extra weight throughout the body, albeit more around the middle. Thus, we were intrigued to find a feasible approach to combat the accumulation of the fat on our body. As a result, we presented a diverse array of diet options to choose from. Since this was an overwhelming bulk, we had to narrow down some more pragmatic alternatives. However, it turns out that there is no one-formula-cures-all version in weight loss battle. Hence, we had to offer a few substitutes that could be practically potent in the expedition. Therefore, what we expect through the whole exploration is that our readers grow the insight to decode the enigma of the weight gain and decide for themselves about the effective strategy to attain the goal of losing the uncomfortable weight.

References

Solan, M. (2022, April 1). *A healthier way to look at body fat*. Harvard Health. https://www.health.harvard.edu/staying-healthy/a-healthier-way-to-look-at-body-fat

Caballero, A. E. (2022, May 24). *Diabetes: Does a long-term study reinforce or change approaches to prevention?* Harvard Health. https://www.health.harvard.edu/blog/diabetes-does-a-long-term-study-reinforce-or-change-approaches-to-prevention-202205242750

Godman, H. (2022, June 1). *Warning: Older age makes you vulnerable to the summer heat*. Harvard Health. https://www.health.harvard.edu/diseases-and-conditions/warning-older-age-makes-you-vulnerable-to-the-summer-heat

Salamon, M. (2022, June 1). *The truth about nutrient deficiencies*. Harvard Health. https://www.health.harvard.edu/nutrition/the-truth-about-nutrient-deficiencies

Salamon, M. (2022, December 1). *Eating disorders in midlife*. Harvard Health. https://www.health.harvard.edu/womens-health/eating-disorders-in-midlife

Salamon, M. (2023, January 1). *Surprising foods that boost bone health*. Harvard Health. https://www.health.harvard.edu/womens-health/surprising-foods-that-boost-bone-health

Salamon, M. (2023, August 1). *Feeding body and soul*. Harvard Health. https://www.health.harvard.edu/nutrition/feeding-body-and-soul

Shaw, G. (2021, March 19). *Losing Weight After 50: Success Stories*. WebMD. https://www.webmd.com/healthy-aging/features/losing-weight-after-fifty

Healthy Meal Planning: Tips for Older Adults. (n.d.). National Institute on Aging. https://www.nia.nih.gov/health/healthy-meal-planning-tips-older-adults

Maintaining a Healthy Weight. (n.d.). National Institute on Aging. https://www.nia.nih.gov/health/maintaining-healthy-weight

4 Secrets to Aging Happily. (2020, December 19). Canyon Ranch. https://www.canyonranch.com/well-stated/post/4-secrets-to-aging-happily/

A Man's Changing Body. (2021, February 18). Canyon Ranch. https://www.canyonranch.com/well-stated/post/a-mans-changing-body/

Healthy Eating Tips for Women, From Your 30s to Your 60s+. (2021, September 4). Canyon Ranch. https://www.canyonranch.com/well-stated/post/women-eating-for-every-stage-of-life/

Downing, D. (2022, November 3). *A Woman's Changing Body*. Canyon Ranch. https://www.canyonranch.com/well-stated/post/a-womans-changing-body/

Pa-C, J. A. G. J. M. (2021, January 7). *Weight Loss for Women Over 50 Is Hard, but This Might Make It Much Harder*. Testosterone Centers of Texas. https://tctmed.com/weight-loss-for-women-over-50/

Lawler, M. (2022, July 12). *5 Reasons It's Harder to Lose Weight With Age and What to Do About It*. EverydayHealth.com. https://www.everydayhealth.com/weight/weight-gain-and-aging.aspx

Farooq, Y. (2022, October 19). *5 Factors That Can Make Weight Loss Harder After 50*. Nutrisense Journal. https://www.nutrisense.io/blog/weight-loss-after-50

Goad, K. (2023, August 23). *20 Expert Tips for Losing Weight After 50*. AARP. https://www.aarp.org/health/healthy-living/info-2021/weight-loss-after-50.html

McCulloch, T. (2020, June 23). *Why is it so hard for women over 50 to lose weight?* Northwest Community Healthcare. https://www.nch.org/news/why-is-it-so-hard-for-women-over-50-to-lose-weight/

Shaw, G. (2021, March 19). *Losing Weight After 50: Success Stories*. WebMD. https://www.webmd.com/healthy-aging/features/losing-weight-after-fifty

Crouch, M. (2023, July 6). *6 Things Women Wish Their Doctors Told Them About Turning 50*. AARP. https://www.aarp.org/health/healthy-living/info-2023/women-turning-50-health-changes.html

What to Expect in Your 50s. (n.d.). WebMD. https://www.webmd.com/healthy-aging/ss/slideshow-what-to-expect-in-your-50s

R, S. (2023, May 19). *Major Changes in Women's Body After 50: Hormonal Shifts & Immune System*. Motherhood Hospitals India. https://www.motherhoodindia.com/what-a-womans-body-experiences-in-their-50s/#:~:text=Hormonal%20Shifts%20and%20Menopause%20Symptoms%20in%20Women%20Over%2050&text=This%20alteration%20can%20lead%20to,also%20becomes%20thinner%20and%20drier